Keto Diet f
Over 50

Discovering Step-by-Step the Secrets to Burn Fat and Lose Weight Quickly, Balance Hormones, Increase Your Energy and Get Young Again with Keto Diet

SOPHIA DAVIES

CONTENTS

Introduction

Congratulations on purchasing Keto Diet for Women Over 50 and starting your journey toward better health and wellness. I am excited for you to begin learning how the ketogenic lifestyle can transform your physical health.

This book is your guide to a new way of thinking about food, energy, fats and carbs, and yes, calories and weight loss. Whatever your health goals, subscribing to a keto diet can unlock a new mindset about the meals you consume and how caloric energy can better serve you. If this sounds complicated, it doesn't need to be! It's science, but it's not rocket science! In these pages, you'll find step-by-step guidance on how to burn fat more efficiently every day while still eating foods you love and stopping the cycle of measuring food or counting calories. Even better, the keto lifestyle allows you to drastically increase your energy levels and reduce a wide array of health risks in the process. You'll find meal plans, recipes, and exercises to add to your keto toolbox, setting you up for the success you deserve.

There are plenty of books on keto diets on the market, many of them designed as one-size-fits-all diet plans. The Keto Diet for Women Over 50 is different. It is targeted to the specific demographic of women 50-plus, addressing the particular ways in which a ketogenic diet works in your body. I am glad you're here, and I hope that as you unlock the easy steps of adopting a keto lifestyle, you will consider leaving a review on Amazon. Your review helps others make the informed choice toward healthier living.

As you begin to plan your keto diet, you will need a way to keep track of your macros, carbs, and calories and a place to organize your keto meal plan and weekly recipes.

In this bundle, you'll receive:

•A Daily Diet Tracker to keep track of the food you eat.

•A Daily Low Carb Tracker to keep track of the carbs you eat and your Carb Target.

•A Weekly Keto Meal Planner. We discussed the benefits of being prepared and having your keto menu planned out ahead of time. You will cheat fewer times and feel tempted less often! Our weekly planner has space for you to write down your keto meals for breakfast, lunch, and dinner every day for each week. Laminate this one-sheet planner and use a dry-erase marker to reuse it week by week, or simply print a new sheet every Sunday!

Here's the link to have these 3 completely free tools, copy it on your favorite device!

https://www.subscribepage.com/ketodiettools

Now let's go back to our Keto Diet.

Let's get started!

Chapter 1: What Is a Keto Diet?

In simplest terms, the ketogenic diet (or keto diet) is a diet focusing on low carbs and high protein. It offers many health benefits. A lot like Atkins and other low-carb diets, a keto diet focuses on lowering your carbohydrate intake by a large amount and replacing this with fat. 'Fat' has a negative connotation for many people but increasing your fat intake is actually necessary on a keto diet because it allows you to enter a metabolic state called ketosis.

As soon as you are in ketosis, your body becomes very good at burning fat for energy. So, what may have seemed like an unintuitive step toward weight loss—adding fat to your diet—actually ends up being a significant benefit. As an added plus, being in ketosis transforms fat into ketones in your liver. Why is this a benefit? Because this process supplies extra energy to the brain.

Dialing Into the Details

To be successful with a keto diet, you first need to understand *why* it works. By understanding the basic nutritional and biological science behind keto, you can make a keto diet work for you in practical ways. So, let's dig into the details.

What Is Ketosis?

Ketosis is a metabolic state. It occurs when your body turns to fat as fuel instead of using carbohydrates. Carbs are essentially glucose (sugar), and normally, glucose is your body's 'go-to' for creating energy. When you significantly reduce or cut carbs out of your diet, you limit the amount of glucose in your body, which means you must get creative and use something else to make energy. What does it use? Fat!

Following a keto diet is the easiest path to ketosis. In the most basic sense, while on keto, you will need to limit your carb consumption to around 20, 30, or 50 grams per day, substituting additional carbs with healthy fats. Examples of healthy fats include meats, fish, eggs, nuts, and healthy oils such as coconut oil or olive oil.

What Is a Ketone, and What Role Does It Play?

You already learned that being in ketosis turns fat into ketones, but what, exactly, is a ketone? Simply put: ketones are byproducts of the breakdown of fat, or fatty acids, in the body. Everyone on any type of diet breaks fat down into fuel, creating ketones in the process. Usually, insulin, glucagon, and other hormones keep the ketone levels from getting too high. Remember: carbs are sugar, and sugar is glucose, and the body turns to glucose to create energy first. So, on an average diet that includes carbs, ketones don't build up in the blood system.

But the magic happens when the body is low on carbs. Carbs, as you might remember, are converted to sugar. When carbs are absent, the ketone levels rise. When this happens, the result is a reduction in blood sugar and insulin levels. Without insulin at the ready to be converted to energy, the body burns fat instead. The burning of this fat creates energy. In this way, you can 'jump start' the fat-burning process by getting your body into ketosis.

How to Know When You've Entered Ketosis

'Entering ketosis' is the goal when you're on a keto diet, as ketosis offers many health benefits, including the efficient burning of fat that we've previously discussed. You can expect many biological changes when you enter ketosis as your blood sugar changes and insulin levels reduce. The increased fat breakdown also results in changes you will note in your body as your liver becomes more efficient at producing ketones.

What are these changes? The following are all signs that you may have entered ketosis. Some are not necessarily positive, but they can still give us a clue as to what our body is going through internally.

- Bad breath: Yes, you're likely to experience bad breath while on a keto diet, no matter how strong your dental hygiene game. Your breath may take on a slightly fruity smell because of the reduction in carbs in your diet.
- Weight loss: You are likely to welcome this symptom that you've entered ketosis more enthusiastically. Weight loss can be expected on a short-term and long-term basis on a keto diet. First to go will be water weight, but most women on a keto diet can expect to continue to lose body fat as long as they are consistent with keto.
- Decreased appetite: This is another welcome change! When in ketosis, your body increases its efficiency at making energy so that you may feel less hungry.
- Better focus: This sign of ketosis is harder to measure, but as your body adapts to burning more fat for fuel, the initial 'keto brain fog' some people report clears up, and increased focus is enjoyed.
- More energy: Along with increased focus, people in ketosis often report having more energy throughout the day. Why? Ketones are an excellent fuel source!
- Short-term fatigue: Remember that mention of 'keto brain fog'? Also known as 'keto flu,'

some people entering ketosis report a temporary lack of energy. This side effect is simply a side effect of weaning yourself off of a carb-heavy diet. Your body must get used to a new normal.

● Short-term decreased performance: If you're an athlete, you may feel a short-term decrease in your normal ability levels along with the fatigue mentioned above. Your muscles' glycogen stores become reduced during ketosis, which tends to be the most efficient fuel source during high-intensity activities and workouts. If you're in an ultra-endurance sport, a keto diet is still beneficial, perhaps even more so, but you may first notice a dip in performance before seeing the rewards.

●Digestive sensitivities: Remember, a keto diet is likely a significant change for your body, and as such, most people can expect some digestive issues or inconveniences during ketosis. Eat low-carb veggies, and remember to keep diversity in your diet instead of sticking to a few low-carb foods you already know you enjoy or can tolerate.

●Insomnia: While rare, some people have reported difficulty sleeping while in ketosis. This issue will subside within a few weeks for most keto diet participants.

Methods of Keto Dieting

There are several basic types of keto diets, some of which are better than others for women over 50. The primary keto diets that are generally accepted and followed include:

- **The standard keto diet (SKD):** Enjoy a high-fat (70%), low-carbohydrate (10%) with medium protein counts (20%)
- **The cyclical keto diet (CKD):** Rev it up on this plan using a cycle-based diet that relies on periods of SKD followed by higher carbohydrate days. The balance is usually five days of SKD followed by two days of higher carb consumption
- **High protein keto diet:** You will find this plan is somewhat similar to SKD, but on a high protein keto diet, you are allowed more protein, changing the ratio to approximately 60% fat, 30-25% protein, and usually less than 10% carbs

For most women over 50, an SKD diet or a high protein diet will be the best option for those who are not exercising to an extreme.

Benefits of a Keto Diet

Many people considering a keto diet are motivated by a weight loss goal. If this is your primary goal, you're in the right place because many studies have shown that participants on a keto diet lose weight, sometimes dramatically. Studies have shown keto to be better for weight loss than a low-fat diet, even if the caloric consumption is similar or the same. Many experts believe this is because of the metabolic advantage a low-carb diet offers, as the body learns to burn fat efficiently. Others attribute the better weight loss success to the natural reduction in appetite, which occurs on a high fat, high protein diet.

Weight loss is most noticeable in the early days of a keto diet, which adds to a feeling of accomplishment and encouragement. If you've ever been on a diet and have not seen any measurable success in the first week or so, you know how discouraging this can feel! On keto, you are most likely to see a significant drop in weight during the first week of your diet. The amount can be anywhere from 2-10 pounds.

So, why does a keto diet work so well? As higher protein intake allows the body to convert fat and protein into carbs for fuel, a process called gluconeogenesis occurs. This process triggers many other positive things to happen in the body. Firstly, the appetite is naturally more suppressed than on a 'regular' diet. You're simply not as hungry when you're focusing on consuming proteins and fats. As a result, you'll start to see changes in your hunger hormones, such as leptin and ghrelin.

You'll also begin to burn more fat during rest than you might on a standard diet consisting of more carbohydrates. Your energy levels will also likely be higher than usual, prompting more daily exercise. In this manner, the benefits of a keto diet build upon one another, all aiding in weight loss, should that be your goal.

The benefits of a keto diet do not stop at weight loss, however. Losing weight is just an (often welcome) side effect of a high protein diet. As the body becomes better at burning energy, the metabolism improves. You can eliminate many risk factors for metabolic diseases when your metabolism becomes more efficient.

For instance, on a keto diet, you will likely benefit from improved insulin sensitivity, which can help increase fuel utilization and jump-start your metabolism. This benefit can lower your risk for type 2 diabetes.

The decreased fat storage in your body may also reduce lipogenesis, which is the process of converting sugar into fat. When there are limited carbs in the body, you will simply burn fat for energy instead!

In addition, ketone bodies, which, as you learned, are molecules produced during ketosis, can help protect against some diseases such as certain cancers, epilepsy, and Alzheimer's.

If you suffer from inflammation, the ketonic diet can drastically reduce this as well, as healthy insulin function can help fight chronic inflammation.

Many risk factors for diabetes and heart disease can be reduced or eliminated on a keto diet. You can reduce or eliminate high blood pressure and increased waist-to-hip ratio (the dreaded belly fat). You can also lower your levels of LDL cholesterol (often referred to as the bad kind) and raise your levels of HDL cholesterol, which is the good kind. You can also lower blood sugar levels.

Why Does Keto Help Reduce The Risk of Diabetes?

Insulin plays a huge role in metabolic diseases such as type 2 diabetes. And as you already learned, ketogenic diets are highly effective at lowering insulin levels. This happens as the body learns to burn fat, instead of sugar, for energy. You can reduce blood sugar spikes with the lowering of carbs consumed. In fact, one study found that after only a few weeks on a keto diet, insulin sensitivity improved to a degree of 75 percent, and blood sugar dropped in the participants. Many of these participants were able to eliminate diabetic medication as a result.

Those with type 2 diabetes on a keto diet should take a few additional precautions. It can be good to test your blood sugar levels. You can test yourself throughout the day to make sure they are within their target range and test your ketone levels if your blood sugar is higher than approximately 240-250 mg/dL. Purchase at-home urine testing strips over-the-counter.

Those with type 2 diabetes will want to watch adding fat to any diet, especially if you have obesity or weight loss is your primary goal. The key is to know what types of fat are keto-friendly and which to avoid. On a keto diet, you still need to avoid saturated fats, a leading contributor to obesity and focus on heart-healthy fats, such as fish, eggs, avocado, and olive oil. We'll dive into specific keto foods and grocery lists in the coming chapters.

Whether you're interested in a keto diet to help manage a metabolic disease, such as diabetes, or to lose weight, you will also reap the benefits of several additional reduced health risks. These benefits can be true for all people, so next, let's dive into what women can expect from a keto diet and women over age 50 in particular.

Chapter 2: Keto for Women Over 50

Subscribing to a keto diet can jump-start weight loss for women over 50, offering the chance for drastic change during a time of life when losing weight can be especially difficult. But to get the most out of a keto lifestyle, it's essential to understand the impact ketosis and a keto diet can have on a women's hormones, fertility, and menopause, especially at age 50 and above.

A keto diet is perfect for women over 50 because a high-fat, low-carb diet naturally aids in reducing many issues women can face during this time of life beyond weight gain, such as heart disease, type 2 diabetes, and in some cases, even Alzheimer's disease. It's a win-win!

When you can burn ketones for fuel, the positive effects absorb throughout the body, increasing your energy levels, reducing inflammation, and aiding in focus and concentration.

If you have a history of yo-yo dieting or just can't seem to stick with any particular diet, keto could be a great choice because instead of restrictions and rules, you are learning to eat differently for a long-term lifestyle. The adjustments to your diet, driven by biology and science, do not include limiting portions. Instead, if you listen to your body, you will be guided by your own decreased appetite and your own lack of dependence on carbs.

Remember, if you're struggling with insulin resistance or have type 2 diabetes, a keto diet can often be a useful way for you to consume calories and gain energy in a way that works with what your body needs.

If you've entered or passed menopause, a keto diet can help your body burn fat most efficiently, reducing the risk of weight gain that can be typical for post-menopausal women.

In short, a keto diet can work as a lifestyle change for just about any woman over 50, especially if these changes can extend to your family, partner, or spouse, and social eating. For instance, as an added benefit of your keto lifestyle, your grandchildren might also become less dependent on carbs, losing any necessary weight along with you. Or your spouse may enjoy lower heart disease risk, or your grown children may learn to have a better relationship with sugar and carbs. The idea is to view keto as a way of life you can maintain long after you have reached your weight loss or health goals.

When you are on a keto diet, it's essential to understand how a high-fat, high-protein diet affects women versus men and women over 50 in particular. We'll also look at how a keto diet affects women experiencing pre-menopause, menopause, and peri-menopause.

How Keto Works in a Woman's Body

If you've ever started a diet—any diet—at the same time as a man (maybe a spouse or friend), you already know the cold, hard truth: men typically lose weight faster than women. It's not fair, but there's science behind it.

We can blame evolution. Whether we like it or not, a women's body is always preparing for a potential pregnancy, so we always have at least 10 percent more fat stored 'just in case' than men do. We also have less muscle built up on average, and since muscle burns more calories than fat, we're already at a disadvantage. It's as if men get a 'head start' when a man and a woman begin a diet simultaneously.

And when we've left our child-bearing years behind us, we still have a disadvantage because menopause naturally adds on pounds as well, especially around the lower abdomen. So, what can women do?

A keto diet may be even more beneficial for women than men because switching from running on carbs to running on fat can even the playing field, even if just a little. As a woman, you'll get to use that extra fat storage to your advantage; as soon as your body realizes that it has the green light to start using that fat to create energy, you'll have ready-made fuel to burn. You can eat fewer calories while knowing your body is turning to that 'reserve' of fat.

How Keto Is Different for Women Than fia or Men

Women have a vast array of considerations about which that men don't have to think. Again, not fair! The first consideration involves hormones. Yes, men have hormones too, but women are more sensitive to dietary changes. Starting a keto diet is a pretty drastic nutritional change, and as a result, you can expect a few noticeable changes to your hormones.

If you have not entered menopause yet, you may experience lower estrogen levels. As you begin a keto diet, you naturally reduce the amount of processed food you consume. Processed food contains a lot of soybean oil, and a sudden lack of this can lower your estrogen. Low estrogen can cause lower sex drive, restless sleep, and some changes to your mood.

However, suppose you are pre-menopausal or have already entered into menopause, as most women over 50 are. In that case, you may instead experience *higher* estrogen levels when you are on a keto diet. Why? Because your estrogen levels have already naturally reduced, and the higher protein intake can increase them. This fact is an excellent added benefit of a keto diet!

A keto diet will also lower your insulin levels, which, as we know, results in less sugar in the body. When sugar is abundant in a woman's body, it blocks weight loss. Therefore, the lower insulin level can help women lose weight faster and easier.

The next consideration for many women on a keto diet is a woman's period. If you're still experiencing a period, cravings for sweets (there's that pesky sugar again!) can increase, making it more challenging to stick to a keto diet. But, don't be discouraged if you get on the scale and don't feel successful during your period. Remember that bloating and water weight are authentic side effects during your period, and the resulting weight gain will only be temporary. Stick with it!

Women also have carb consumption to consider more than men. While on a keto diet, it's crucial to reduce carbs, but women must be careful not to reduce them to too extreme of a level, or they risk their body going into 'starvation mode,' in which the female body shuts down fat-burning and tries to 'store it' as an emergency attempt at survival.

What can women do about this? Adding just a *bit* more carbs than men can signal to your body that everything is okay, giving it the go-ahead to burn fat. And keep in mind that as a woman, you'll want to add a few more carbs if you are exercising extensively, bodybuilding, or in a perimenopausal or menopausal stage.

The next consideration has more to do with how women typically view dieting or have historically been educated about dieting than it does about the female body. What am I talking about here? The 'fat consumption' myth. As women, we're typically told not to eat too much fat, and many diets focus heavily on reducing fat or picking 'low-fat' or 'fat-free' options. On a keto diet, we need to embrace fat in our daily food intake! We cannot shy away from fats, because as women, fat is our friend.

While on a keto diet, the higher intake of protein and fat can make women feel fuller, and when we feel full, we consume fewer calories. This benefit is great, but it's important to remember to eat enough! Yes, while following a keto diet, you may have to remind yourself to eat!

Cultural expectations are at the heart of the next consideration that applies more typically to women than most men. In many households, women prepare more family meals than men. And therefore, mealtimes can be challenging for women on a keto diet. If you're preparing non-keto meals for family members, it can be hard to avoid that pizza crust or that dinner roll. The best strategy for women on a keto diet: make it a family affair. Start by identifying your family's favorite meals, then look for ways to make these meals keto-friendly. There are many websites, cookbooks, and apps to help you on this mission. Or, if you typically make most of the meals in the household, perhaps use this diet as an opportunity to reimagine the cultural norms you subscribe to if you choose to do so.

Keto Diet and Menopause

If you're experiencing menopause or pre-menopause as a woman over age 50, you know that it can be especially hard to lose weight during this time of your life. Hormones play a major role in how fat is stored in the body, and as we know, hormones are a bit out of control during menopause. As hormones decrease, more fat becomes stored in the body (thanks, body!). This fat is usually focused on the belly, whereas before menopause, women experience fat stored in the breasts, thighs, and hips.

There's hope! In addition to helping kick start weight loss during a time of life when weight loss is difficult, a keto diet can offer added benefits specifically to menopausal women. The low-carb lifestyle prompts the lowering of insulin and improves insulin sensitivity, which can keep you from feeling too hungry. It can also keep hot flashes at bay, which is a huge added plus!

Women over 50 on a keto diet have reduced their heart disease risk, which is especially beneficial after the natural reduction of estrogen during menopause. Take the following example under consideration. One keto dieter—we'll call her Dana—struggled for years with weight gain, high cholesterol, and autoimmune disorders. After beginning a keto diet at age 65, she lost 40 pounds and now better manages her heart health and autoimmune issues.

Dana is only one of many, many case study examples, and while results—of course—vary, women over 50 do very well on a high protein, low carb diet program. Remember, keto-friendly foods can make you feel fuller, which in turn reduces calorie intake. During a time of life when it's very easy to gain weight without trying, a keto diet as a long-term lifestyle can help keep weight loss on track.

And for women over 50 who have struggled with dieting for years, or maybe even decades, a keto lifestyle can stop that yo-yo dieting habit. Instead of confusing the body with multiple approaches for short-term success, the female body can lean into the consistency offered by a keto diet. Think of keto as a way of being, a form of eating, and a lifestyle, and health gains are sure to follow.

Keto Strategies Specifically for Women Over 50

Women over 50 need a little more time than men to adjust to a keto diet. Like I mentioned, starting too quickly can 'panic' the body, sending it into fat storage mode. Therefore, women starting a keto diet should limit their carbs slowly.

Start by tracking how many carbs you consume on a daily basis on your average diet. Maybe you're in the typical range of 250-300 grams of carbs per day. From that benchmark, you can make a plan to adjust your carb intake gradually until you're at the recommended ten percentage.

Some good news: studies have shown that most women find weight loss success on a keto diet without reducing carb intake to the maximum. For example, when 24 women followed a low-carb diet for eight weeks, they experienced an average of 20 pounds each of weight loss. They also reduced their blood sugar levels, insulin resistance, and free testosterone levels by limiting their carbs to approximately 70 grams per day, compared to the 25 grams per day required by men.

We'll get into a detailed keto diet 'game plan' for women in the following chapters, but for now, just know that your carb reduction will be a gradual process, and there's science behind this. This gradual reduction allows your body to adjust and adapt naturally to the change and 'believe' that yes, it can get by on fewer carbs. You and your body will learn this together!

And what about those other disadvantages women face? It's possible to curb period cravings on a keto diet with the right snacks, which I will detail soon. Women can also do well when adding resistance training to their exercise routine to help continue to hone those muscles as the body turns to them to create energy. We'll outline specific exercises for women on a keto diet in the coming chapter.

Women will also be successful on a keto diet by tracking food intake and keeping a keto journal. We'll show you how to do this, as well as point you in the direction of the many helpful keto diet apps and programs available to you. In your keto journal, you'll measure both tangible and intangible successes, such as weight loss, inches lost, mood enhancement, increased energy, and cravings.

When a Keto Diet May Not Be Suitable for You

Most, in fact, almost all women over 50 can experience great success with a keto diet. There are some exceptions, however, for women who experience any of the following factors. These women need to ask a physician before pursuing a keto diet. These factors can include:

- Women who have liver failure or kidney failure
- Women who have alcohol or drug use disorders
- Those with type 1 diabetes
- Those who have pancreatitis
- Women with disorders that affect fat metabolism
- Those with carnitine deficiency
- Women who have trouble with adequate nutritional intake
- Women with porphyria

Ready to learn more? It's time to get into the nitty-gritty of a keto diet and how to make a keto lifestyle work for you.

Specific Health Benefits of Keto for Women 50+

We've discussed the many health benefits available to both men and women on a keto diet, but some added benefits affect older women more than any other demographic.

Better Bone Health and Lower Osteoporosis Risk

Osteoporosis is a condition in which reduced bone density results in bones becoming fragile and breaking easily and is very common in older women. Conventional wisdom has long prescribed more calcium for women over 50 to combat osteoporosis; however, studies have shown that countries with high rates of osteoporosis also tend to have the highest rates of dairy consumption. Instead, a keto diet can be best for preventing brittle bones because it is naturally low in toxins, which interfere with the absorption of nutrients. A keto diet is plentiful in all micronutrients, not just dairy.

Fewer Nutrient Deficiencies

Older women are often deficient in some nutrients, such as iron, vitamin B12, vitamin D, and heart-healthy fats. These deficiencies can lead to fatigue, brain 'fog,' neurological conditions such as dementia, skin and vision problems, cancer, and heart disease. There's a reason your primary care provider is probably adding these supplements to your diet! But women can eliminate taking so many costly vitamins and supplements by focusing instead on be deliberate with a keto diet.

Controlling Blood Sugar

Let's face it: it's a lot harder to live off of processed food and fast food after age 50 than when you were a teenager. Somehow, those calories don't just magically disappear like they used to. The fact is, women over 50 have to be more careful about everything they put in their bodies. While on a keto diet or keto lifestyle, the lowered intake of carbohydrates, especially from processed foods with high fructose or high saturated fats, results in lower blood sugar. Lower blood sugar results in the reduction of those neurological diseases we previously discussed, such as dementia, Alzheimer's, and even Parkinson's disease.

Keto-friendly foods deliver higher nutrition per calorie. And as older adults, we want to pack more punch into each calorie because our bodies require fewer of them than when we were younger. In other words, no more empty calories. Each calorie needs to count!

Increased Hormonal Balance

Menopause or no, women over 50 can expect just about anything when it comes to their hormones. One day everything seems 'normal,' and then next, everything seems to have shifted out of our control. As we deal with the side effects of menopause, it becomes more important than ever to find hormonal balance. A keto diet helps maintain this balance as it minimizes simple carbs and sugar while upping the intake of heart-healthy fats. Just be sure not to jump-start keto too drastically (instead easing into a keto diet), or you may risk triggering your cortisol hormone, also known as your stress hormone. Remember, women can find success on keto without reducing carbs too drastically.

The earlier in life you decide to make a positive change for yourself and adopt a keto lifestyle, the earlier you can improve your immunity, blood sugar levels, and neurological health. The sooner you will have the energy to enjoy more of what life offers at a healthy weight.

Time to get started!

Chapter 3: the Nice and Naughty List (Keto-Friendly Foods and Foods To Avoid)

Any dietary plan needs structure. If you've ever followed a diet 'halfway' or adopted a moderate approach to controlling what you eat without parameters, you know that it can be easy to 'fall off the wagon.' A keto lifestyle does not have unbendable 'rules' to follow, but the science behind a keto diet does give us a road map for success.

Before you can create a keto meal plan and start mapping out your first few weeks of keto, you need to know what, exactly, should go on your grocery shopping list. What is considered a high-carb food? For that matter, what foods should you definitely avoid, and what foods should you always embrace? Let's get into the details.

What, Exactly, Are Keto-Friendly Foods?

You now already know that keto-approved foods tend to be much higher in protein or fat and lower in carbs. Many resources exist to help steer you toward these foods, and I will suggest some of these resources in our lists of favorite keto tools and tricks. But for now, let's get a basic overview of keto-friendly foods, divided into subgroups.

Fish and Seafood

Why? Fish is protein-rich and carbohydrate-free, and it is also rich in B vitamins, potassium, and selenium. Great choices for your keto diet include salmon, sardines, mackerel, and albacore tuna, as these are all fatty fish choices with high levels of omega-3 fats (these fats can lower your blood sugar levels and even raise your insulin sensitivity). Shellfish are also on the approved list, as shrimp and crab have no carbs at all, but note that other shellfish, such as oysters, clams, and mussels, can contain more carbs than most fatty fish.

Fish and Seafood Complete List

- Salmon
- Sardines
- Mackerel
- Shellfish
- Tuna
- Octopus

- Squid
- Cod
- Halibut
- Swordfish
- Mahi Mahi
- Flounder

Low-Carb Vegetables

Be careful here because not all veggies are on the nice list! It helps to remember to go green. Examples of low-carb veggies include green, leafy vegetables, broccoli, cauliflower, green beans, peppers, zucchini, and spinach. Many of these veggies also contain high amounts of fiber, and most keto carb counters agree that when counting carbs, you can subtract fiber from carbs to get a 'net carb' amount (carbs minus fiber).

Consume veggies like cauliflower, green kale, and broccoli, linked to a decrease in some cancers and heart disease, without restriction. The key is to avoid starchy veggies, such as potatoes, most squashes, and corn.

Vegetable Complete List

- Asparagus
- Avocado
- Broccoli

- Cabbage
- Cauliflower
- Cucumber
- Eggplant
- Green beans
- Kale
- Leafy green lettuce
- Mushrooms
- Olives
- Peppers
- Spinach
- Tomatoes
- Zucchini

Dairy

Yes, cheese is on the nice list! Don't go crazy with dairy, but you have the green light to eat cheese, heavy cream, milk, and yogurt on the keto diet. Just remember that while rich in protein and calcium, dairy also delivers saturated fats. This unfortunate fact is especially true for cheese. Cottage cheese is a good pick, as is unsweetened yogurt. Five ounces of plain Greek yogurt only has five grams of carbohydrates yet packs 18 grams of protein.

Cheese Complete List

- Blue cheese
- Brie
- Camembert
- Cheddar
- Chevre
- Colby jack
- Cottage cheese
- Cream cheese
- Crumbled feta
- Goat cheese
- Havarti
- Limburger
- Manchego
- Mozzarella
- Parmesan cheese
- Pepper jack
- Provolone
- Romano
- Swiss
- String cheese

Additional Dairy Complete List

- Heavy cream
- Sour cream
- Unsweetened yogurt

- Unsweetened Greek yogurt
- Butter
- Mayonnaise

Some Fruit

As some keto diet enthusiasts will tell you to avoid all fruit on a keto diet, this one is controversial. For women over 50, some fruit may be beneficial, as it allows for a more gentle transition into a low-carb diet, as discussed earlier. The best fruit to include in your keto diet includes berries, especially raspberries and avocado. Avocado is an especially keto-friendly food, so you'll see many keto recipes that include avocado. It's a heart-healthy fat option with nine grams of carbs, but seven of these grams are fiber. Avocado oil, along with other plant-based oils and fats, is an excellent option to replace animal fats if you're concerned about cholesterol levels and triglyceride levels.

Avoid sugar-heavy fruit. These include 'juicy' fruits such as apples, oranges, grapes, and melons. Bananas pack quite a bit of sugar, too.

Fruit Complete List

- Blackberries
- Blueberries
- Raspberries
- Strawberries

- Avocado

Meat and Poultry

You probably already know that a keto diet can consist of plenty of animal fats and meats. Meat can be a great source of leaner proteins and has zero carbs. You also get plenty of minerals and B vitamins from meat and poultry. However, try to limit the number of processed meats you eat on keto. These can include sausage and bacon, as too much can be bad for your cholesterol levels and heart. You'll also want to read the ingredient labels on processed deli meats to avoid sugar. Otherwise, you have a green light for meat and poultry!

Meat and Poultry Complete List

- Lean beef
- Chicken
- Lamb
- Goat
- Pork
- Eggs

Eggs

Eggs get their own category. For many people, eggs are another staple on a keto diet, as they can work in many recipes and adapt to many meals. Hard-boiled eggs are an excellent option to add to any keto lunch, and of course, eggs at breakfast are an easy pick. Like meat, eggs have no carbs yet have 12 grams of protein. They also pack B vitamins and antioxidants. As an added bonus, eggs can help make you feel full.

Coffee and Tea

You may be bidding goodbye to your favorite alcoholic beverages on a keto diet, but you are good to go with coffees and teas. The only catch: you need to drink them unsweetened. Opt for a creamer that's unflavored or flavored without sugar, and coffee lowers the risk of cardiovascular disease and type 2 diabetes. Studies have also shown many teas to reduce the risk of a heart attack. Tea drinking can also help with weight loss and even lower the risk of stroke in some people.

Tip: Remember that you can also enjoy sparkling waters, even the flavored variety, provided they do not contain any added sugar.

Nuts, Seeds, and Oils

Nuts, seeds, and oils are a big category! Feel free to go nuts with nuts! Again, you'll need to remember to reach for the unsweetened variety, which means avoiding the more processed options like honey-roasted or candied. Peanut butter is a go if unsweetened, so again, read the labels. Almond butter is a great option, as are many seed blends, such as those found in grain-free granola mixes.

Nuts contain some carbohydrates, so bear this in mind when choosing which type you want to add to your diet. Brazil nuts, walnuts, and pecans have the least amount of carbs, while almonds, cashews, and pistachios contain more. Still, all are under five grams per serving. The best seeds to reach for include chia seeds (these do a great job of helping you feel full, too) and flaxseeds, which have no carbs at all. Pumpkin seeds are also a good bet.

Animal fats and oils are okay to consume on a keto diet, but even better are plant-based oils. Look to avocado oil, but even more so to coconut oil and olive oil. Coconut oil is a great choice when you are craving a little sweetness to your diet. Remember that it's high in saturated fats, but it's also bursting with triglycerides, known to boost ketone production.

Nuts, Seeds, and Oils Complete List

- Walnuts
- Brazil nuts
- Almonds
- Cashews

- Pecans
- Macadamia nuts
- Pistachios
- Flaxseed
- Chia seeds
- Pumpkin seeds
- Sunflower seeds
- Sesame seeds

Condiments and Dressings

You're going to want to dress up those leafy green salads and marinate that fatty fish, and the good news is, many condiments and dressings are on the nice list. The main rule of thumb: make sure you avoid dressings that contain sugar.

Condiments and Dressings Complete List

- Balsamic vinegar
- Mayonnaise
- Mustard
- Unsweetened ketchup
- Coconut aminos
- Hot sauce
- Sugar-free steak sauce
- Homemade ranch dressing
- Italian vinaigrette
- Marinara sauce
- Green goddess dressing

• Yogurt-based dressings

Dark Chocolate

Okay, but what about dessert? Yes, you can eat chocolate on keto! Here's the catch: it needs to be dark chocolate or cocoa powder, as these foods are considered superfoods. Dark chocolate is higher than most foods in antioxidants, and therefore, chocolate can lower your blood pressure and even lower your risk of heart disease. Go, chocolate!

Foods to Avoid On Keto

Now that you know what you *can* eat, it's reasonably intuitive to understand what you must avoid. The easy way to stick to your keto diet is to find a cheat sheet you like (which I will cover in the next chapter) and adhere to the list. But it's also helpful to see the bigger picture. Let's break it down.

The number one rule to remember regarding foods to avoid is—yes, you already know the answer—low carbs. This fact means you must avoid bread, grains, pasta, and potatoes more than any other foods. Here's the complete list of 'no go' foods.

Grains and Grain-Based Foods

- Wheat
- Corn
- Pasta
- Rice
- Granola (made with grains)
- Oats
- Cereal
- Crackers
- Graham crackers
- Quinoa
- Couscous

Sugar-Related Products

- Table sugar
- Honey
- Agave
- Maple syrup
- Soda
- Sports drinks
- Sweetened creamers
- Candy
- Processed snacks
- Granola bars and other energy bars made with sugar
- Most fruit (apples, bananas, oranges, melons, grapes)

- Cocktails
- Sugar-based sweeteners
- Condiments with sugar like ketchup, barbeque sauce, and sugary marinades
- Dressings made with sugar or sugar substitutes
- Soy sauce

Starchy Vegetables

- Potatoes
- French fries
- Yams
- Most squashes
- Sweet potatoes
- Chips

Oils and Fats

- Margarine
- Partially and fully hydrogenated oils
  Oils including:
- Vegetable
- Soybean
- Peanut
- Canola
- Foods cooked in these oils

Dairy

- Cow's milk (especially reduced-fat milk)
- Ice cream

Are There Any Foods on The 'Maybe' List?

Yes, some foods will fall into a 'maybe' or 'sometimes' category. These are foods that may have some net carbs but provide many other benefits for your health. Add or eliminate these foods based on your personal preferences or health needs.

Legumes and Beans

Beans and legumes can be controversial. Who knew? While considered healthy overall, beans do contain carbs. However, their net carb amount is fairly low (remember, you can calculate net carbs by subtracting carbs from fiber in any food). The bottom line: if beans and legumes are essential to your diet, you'll have to decide *how* important. In other words, how many net carbs are you willing to 'spend' on beans?

Tip: if you are trying for a strict keto diet, stick with green beans or black soybeans.

Legumes and Beans Complete List

- Black beans, 12 grams net carbs
- Navy beans, 14 grams net carbs
- Kidney beans, 13 grams net carbs
- Black soybeans, 2 grams net carbs
- Green beans, 2 grams net carbs
- Chickpeas, 18 grams net carbs
- Lima beans, 12 grams net carbs
- Pinto beans, 15 grams net carbs
- Lentils, 11 grams net carbs
- Black-eyed peas, 15 grams net carbs
- Great northern beans, 13 grams net carbs

Alcohol

Purists to a keto diet may shun all alcoholic beverages, but there's good news for those who wish to imbibe moderately. Pure forms of alcohol are carb-free, and many light beers and wines are low on carbs. Just like I mentioned in the section on beans and legumes, individuals who want to consume alcohol will have to decide how much of the daily allotment of carbs will go to that drink. Just remember that using mixers usually results in adding sugar, so avoid cocktails.

Alcohol Complete List

- Rum, 0 grams carbs
- Vodka, 0 grams carbs
- Gin, 0 grams carbs
- Tequila, 0 grams carbs
- Whiskey, 0 grams carbs
- Red wine, 3-4 grams carbs
- White wine, 3-4 grams carbs
- Light beer, 3 grams carbs

Stay away from cocktail mixers such as soda, juice, simple sugar, and sugary energy beverages. Instead, use mixers such as sparkling water or seltzer, club soda without sugar, or sugar-free diet soda (though not advised).

Keto-Friendly Snack Ideas

The food lists in this chapter serve as the groundwork for grocery shopping and meal preparation (covered in Chapter 4).

Most packaged foods are NOT keto-friendly. Therefore, if it's in a package that you have to open, it's probably on the no-go list. Hey, at least it's easy to remember what you can and cannot eat! But the good news is that keto-friendly snacks can be easy to prepare and will be healthier whole food options.

Try any of the following keto snack ideas:

- Sliced cheese and (sugar-free) meats
- Olive and nut medley
- Hard-boiled eggs
- String cheese
- Deviled eggs
- Cucumber sticks and yogurt dip
- Celery and sugar-free peanut or almond butter
- Sweet peppers and Green Goddess dressing
- Veggies and spinach dip
- Berries and heavy cream
- Beef jerky
- Dark chocolate
- Dehydrated kale chips
- Rolled salami and cheese
- Meat bars
- Coconut chips
- Dark chocolate, nut, and berry trail mix
- Pork rinds

When you have a little more time to prepare your keto snacks, look for specific keto snack recipes in the following chapters. You'll stick to your keto goals, and in the process, you'll enjoy more wholesome whole food choices.

How to Use This Nice and Naughty Food List for Best Results

Most keto diet followers aim for 25-50 carbs per day (more on this in the following chapter). How strictly you decide to follow your diet is up to you. Take in mind your health needs and requirements, as well as any goals to lose weight. You can get results from following a general guideline or a firm list to anywhere in-between.

Sometimes, no matter your philosophy, you may find yourself in a situation in which you're just not sure if a food is approved, or you are in a situation lacking keto-friendly options. Maybe you're out to dinner and the restaurant picked is less than keto-friendly, Or perhaps you find yourself stuck in a car all day, carting kids to activities and sports. Maybe you're at work longer than planned, and your planned and prepared keto dinner is waiting at home, uneaten and neglected. Life happens!

When this occurs, simply remember the following fundamental principle:

For every food you eat, you must consider its:

- Net carbs
- Protein and fat content
- Health benefits

You will stay on course for your keto diet if the food in question helps you stay within your daily carb limit, meets your needs for protein and fat, and improves your health and overall sense of wellbeing.

That's it!

And if you have a difficult day, keep in mind that each new day is a brand new chance to do well. When you are consistent over a more extended period, success follows. This keto journey is a lifestyle change, not a short-term diet. A successful keto diet is a marathon, not a sprint!

Chapter 4: Creating a Keto Meal Plan

If you've embarked on diets in the past, you know that planning ahead is critical. It's always easiest to slip in your efforts when you don't have healthy choices ready to go. Before starting on your keto journey, you will want to stock your fridge and cupboards with keto-friendly foods and have keto meal plans on hand. If you're not just cooking for one, decide ahead of time whether these additional housemates or family members will be joining you on keto or whether you will need to accommodate additional dietary needs.

Tip: If you have family members who do not want to join you on keto, many successful keto dieters compromise by keeping non-keto foods and snacks on hand in a separate location, such as a special drawer in the kitchen for snacks and a dedicated shelf in the pantry for staples. Make sure to store your keto-friendly ingredients at the forefront, keeping non-keto foods as 'out of sight, out of mind' as possible.

It can be hard on your mental game and willpower to prepare two evening meals—one keto and one non-keto—so many keto subscribers who are the primary cook in their family invite their family members to join them in a keto evening meal (keeping their non-keto breakfasts and lunches separate). You might not even need to tell them they're eating a keto dinner! Very few people feel 'cheated' or like their meals are 'lacking' on keto since you can fill their plates with plenty of proteins and veggies.

Keto Goals: How to Find the Correct Net Carb to Fat and Protein Balance for Your Keto Needs

To experience success on a keto plan, you must be familiar with your daily benchmark. This is the first step! The exact number of net carbs you will want to consume in a day varies slightly by the person. Let's start with the generalities. The typical keto diet requires the consumption of less than 50-60 grams of net carbs every day. To better visualize this amount, it's less than what you would find in one bagel or one muffin. Some keto dieters aim for as low as 20-25 grams of carbs every day.

Tip: Always keep in mind that a keto diet does not mean eating zero carbs per day! No one should eliminate all carbs all the time.

Whatever exact amount is best for you, the standard ratio you want to aim for is 70-80 percent fat from daily calories, 5-10 percent carbohydrates, and 10-20 percent protein.

As I covered previously, women have a more challenging time losing weight than men, and women over 50 often have the added challenge of going through menopause. Many women in this age group benefit from easing into their keto diet to avoid sending their bodies into 'survival mode.' A woman's body typically tries to conserve fat as an evolutionary survival mechanism. If you wish to try this technique, start with a higher amount of carbs per day, and lower this amount each week until you are at your carb consumption goal.

So, how do you know what *your* exact ratio should be? Answer the following:

- **How often do you exercise?** If you exercise 4-5 times per week, moderately to strenuously, you will be able to eat more carbohydrates and still stay in ketosis.
- **How much weight do you think you want to lose?** If you are obese or are overweight, you will need to eat fewer carbs to stay in ketosis.
- **Do you have a metabolism that you have noted to slow down significantly following menopause?** If so, you may want to start slow and build up (or down, instead!) to the ideal number of net carbs per day.

Keto Versus Other Lifestyle and Short-Term Diets

On a keto diet, you do not need to restrict your portion sizes to the degree required during a typical diet. Trust me, it's not necessary to count every calorie, but you do need to keep your carb portions small, as you *will* be counting carbs. You also need to ensure you are eating enough protein to stay healthy and well-balanced. There are many useful tools and apps which can help make carb counting easier, which we will dive into together in a moment.

Weigh-Ins on Keto

You will also not need to weigh yourself every day on a keto diet. In fact, most keto diet experts recommend weighing yourself only once per week at the maximum. Many keto dieters step onto the scale even less frequently. Day-to-day weigh-ins can very easily lead to discouragement, especially for women. Why is this? Women's weight fluctuates quite dramatically at times due to a woman's cycle, bloating, and water weight.

Instead of weighing yourself often, regularly note how your clothing feels. Fitting properly into your clothing is a better way to measure success on keto.

For instance, if you have pants that used to be tight and now fit or are even baggy, it should be even more cause for celebration than a number moving down on the scale.

Cheat Days on Keto

Should you allow yourself cheat days on keto? Most diets allow for cheat days, during which you can allow yourself a treat or two (or three!). On keto, you run the risk of breaking ketosis if you cheat. Very few studies exist on the risks or negatives of going in and out of ketosis often, but it's vital to stay consistently in ketosis to lose weight and lose inches. If you must allow yourself cheat days, be sure they are not frequent. No 'cheat foods' daily, for instance, and no 'cheat weekends.' Instead, opt for one cheat day less than once per week.

Duration of Keto

Unlike many diets that come and go, most keto subscribers do not stop doing keto once they've met their goals. Instead, keto can become a way of life, perhaps at a moderate level. This practice helps ensure you do not gain the weight back but instead adopt a modified keto diet as a way of life.

Keto Carb and Protein Cheat Sheet

The following list is a helpful tool to help you get a sense of the number of net carbs, fat, and protein in some popular keto foods. This list does not include every possible food you are allowed to eat on a keto diet, but it will be a reference for you as you go forward.

Avocado Oil: 1 t. Serving

124 calories, 14 g fat, 0 net carbs, 0 g protein

Coconut Oil: 1 t. Serving

116 calories, 14 g fat, 0 net carbs, 0 g protein

Butter: 1 t. Serving

100 calories, 11 g fat, 0 net carbs, 0 g protein

Cheddar Cheese: 1 Slice Serving

113 calories, 9 g fat, 0 net carbs, 7 g protein

Heavy Cream: 1 t. Serving

52 calories, 5 g fat, 0 net carbs, 0 g protein

Bacon: 1 Slice per Serving

43 calories, 3 g fat, 0 net carbs, 3 g protein

Chicken Thigh: 1 Thigh per Serving

310 calories, 20 g fat, 0 net carbs, 32 g protein

Eggs: 1 Egg per Serving

77 calories, 5 g fat, 1 net carb, 6 g protein

Ground Beef: 3 oz. Serving

277 calories, 24 g fat, 0 net carbs, 12 g protein

Steak: 3 oz. Serving

225 calories, 14 g fat, 0 net carbs, 22 g protein

Asparagus: 1 c Serving

27 calories, 0 g fat, 2 net carbs, 3 g protein

Avocado: ½ Avocado Serving

160 calories, 15 g fat, 2 net carbs, 2 g protein

Bok Choy: 1 c Serving

9 calories, 0 g fat, 1 net carb, 1 g protein

Cauliflower: 1 c Serving

29 calories, 0 g fat, 2 net carbs, 2 g protein

Celery: 1 c Serving

16 calories, 0 g fat, 1 net carb, 1 g protein

Cucumber: ½ c Serving

8 calories, 0 g fat, 2 net carbs, 0 g protein

Green Peppers: 1 c Serving

6 calories, 0 g fat, 2 net carbs, 1 g protein

Lettuce: 5 c Serving

5 calories, 0 g fat, 1 net carb, 0 g protein

Mushrooms: 1 c Serving

14 calories, 0 g fat, 1 net carb, 2 g protein

Zucchini: 1 c Serving

18 calories, 0 g fat, 3 net carbs, 1 g protein

Sample Two-Week Keto Meal Plan

I talked about making a plan and having your keto-friendly foods ready before you begin your keto diet. The act of sitting down and planning your keto meals can help you get into the right mindset for success and even get you excited to begin your keto journey! Feel free to use the following sample two-week keto meal plan just as it's written or use it as a guideline or inspiration for your keto plan.

Day 1

Breakfast: scrambled eggs cooked in butter topped with avocado slices
Morning snack: mixed nuts
Lunch: mixed green salad with grilled skinless chicken breast and balsamic dressing
Afternoon snack: carrot sticks and Greek yogurt dip
Dinner: air fried salmon with an amino glaze and grilled asparagus in butter

Day 2

Breakfast: Greek yogurt topped with berries
Morning snack: beef jerky
Lunch: tuna salad with mayonnaise topped with sliced tomato on a bed of lettuce
Afternoon snack: cheese slices
Dinner: pork chops with green beans roasted with olive oil

Day 3

Breakfast: cheese omelet topped with avocado, red onion, sour cream, and salsa
Morning snack: hard-boiled egg with salt
Lunch: meat and cheese charcuterie with nuts and olives
Afternoon snack: sugar-free almond butter

Dinner: sashimi and veggie stir fry with tofu

Day 4

Breakfast: almond milk and almond butter protein smoothie
Morning snack: yogurt and grain-free granola
Lunch: fish 'sticks' made with almond flour
Afternoon snack: celery and sugar-free peanut butter
Dinner: roasted chicken with spinach and kale salad

Day 5

Breakfast: fried eggs and bacon
Morning snack: string cheese
Lunch: a burger in a lettuce bun
Afternoon snack: a handful of walnuts and berries
Dinner: halibut baked in a buttercream sauce with broccoli

Day 6

Breakfast: egg 'bites' with peppers and green onion
Morning snack: kale chips
Lunch: seaweed-wrapped salmon and avocado roll-ups
Afternoon snack: meat bar (pork, buffalo, or chicken)
Dinner: chicken kebabs made with onion, peppers, and cauliflower

Day 7

Breakfast: sausage and green pepper omelet
Morning snack: kalamata olives
Lunch: sautéed shrimp with veggie medley
Afternoon snack: turkey jerky
Dinner: New York strip steak with cauliflower 'mash' and butter

Day 8

Breakfast: cashew butter protein shake
Morning snack: berries and cream
Lunch: chicken 'nuggets' made with coconut flour
Afternoon snack: sliced cheese and salami
Dinner: lamb chops with creamed spinach

Day 9

Breakfast: yogurt parfait with chopped nuts and blackberries
Morning snack: hard-boiled eggs
Lunch: chicken salad with mayo over fresh spinach
Afternoon snack: beef sticks
Dinner: salmon filets with a mixed green salad

Day 10

Breakfast: Mexican scramble with avocado, egg, cheese, and salsa

Morning snack: protein smoothie
Lunch: Greek salad with feta, cucumber, and red onion
Afternoon snack: olives and cheese
Dinner: carnitas with cheese, guacamole, and sour cream

Day 11

Breakfast: berry blend smoothie
Morning snack: poached egg
Lunch: chicken drumsticks
Afternoon snack: celery with peanut butter
Dinner: garlic chicken with cauliflower rice

Day 12

Breakfast: bacon and eggs
Morning snack: sliced cucumber and Greek yogurt dip
Lunch: smoked salmon salad
Afternoon snack: Caprese skewers with tomato, mozzarella cheese, and basil
Dinner: turkey stuffed peppers

Day 13

Breakfast: egg cups with cheddar cheese and peppers
Morning snack: kale chips with olives
Lunch: shrimp stir fry on cauliflower rice

Afternoon snack: cheese and meat charcuterie
Dinner: BLT wraps

Day 14

Breakfast: scrambled eggs with salsa and sour cream
Morning snack: mixed nuts and hard-boiled eggs
Lunch: hot dogs with veggies
Afternoon snack: veggie slices with homemade ranch dressing (sugar-free)
Dinner: crispy chicken thighs with roasted Brussel sprouts

Tools and Tips for Keto Meal Planning Success

It's now time to create a keto meal plan for yourself, customized to your preferences. This is the fun part, where you can get excited about the many keto-friendly foods available to you! Many tools and aids exist to assist you in creating your plan, many of which are free resources. If you are on a budget, it's easy to plan your keto meals yourself. If you can splurge a little, you will find additional aids that can certainly make your keto journey easier. It's up to you!

Keto Meal Plan Template

Keep track of your food and customize your keto meal plan with my customizable daily keto log, which you'll find at the end of this book. Simply download the template and populate it with your meal plan choices. Print it and display it somewhere; you will be able to see it and refer to it easily. The best locations to display your meal plans are usually in your kitchen, on the fridge, or inside a cupboard or pantry door.

It can help to laminate your keto meal plans. You can even laminate blank templates and use a dry erase marker to fill in your week's menu. If you will be embarking on your keto journey with your family, allow other family members to contribute meal ideas or add to your keto meal plan as well. A keto diet can be a group project! The more invested everyone is in the keto process, the higher the rate of success.

You may also want to print up a shortlist of non-keto-friendly foods from our list in the previous chapter, which you can also laminate and keep handy in your bag, purse, or pocket. This list is a valuable tool when you find yourself at a loss as to what to order while dining out or what to purchase while at the grocery store. We will have additional tips for keto success while out and about in a later chapter.

Subscription Boxes

Meal subscription services provide all the ingredients for meals delivered directly to your door. For most plans, you first subscribe to the plan, then log onto an app or website to choose your meals weekly or monthly. Many meal subscription services, such as Green Chef, offer keto-specific meal plans. If you're unsure whether your subscription service offers keto meals, check the FAQ section or peruse their page of upcoming meal choices to 'audit' for keto-friendliness yourself.

If your budget allows, opting for meal services with keto recipes can be the easiest way to plan your keto meals for the week.

Alternatively, many additional website services offer pre-set and customized keto meal plans generated for you for a fee. These services do not include the ingredients for your meals but rather only the plan you can download.

While convenient to opt into a paid service for a keto meal plan, this book will give you all the tools you need to plan your meals yourself for free.

Planning, Planning, Planning

Use the keto recipes at the end of this book to create your keto meal plans. Planning your keto meals is a great way to get excited about your week of keto eating, and choosing your recipes can help you feel more invested in the keto diet. Picking and choosing meals yourself can also help ensure that your family members will enjoy the keto recipes you prepare as well.

Keto Macro Calculator

What is a macro? This word is short for macronutrients, which are an essential tool for a keto diet. Think of your keto meal plan this way: your carb intake is a 'limit' (you are limited to a set amount, between 20-50 grams per day once you've eased into ketosis), your protein intake is a 'goal' (you want to reach your protein goal every day), and your fats are a 'lever' (the intake of fats consists of your remaining calories per day after you limit your carbs and reach your protein goal). Fats keep you satisfied and feeling full. Increase your fats if you find you are hungry too often. Decrease fats to lose weight. Just remember you can't go too low, or your body will exit ketosis.

In order to determine just what these numbers should be, then keep track of these numbers, a keto macro calculator can be helpful. You can find one in our list of resources. It determines how much of each type of macronutrients you should consume per day. To use one of the many free macro calculators available online, you only need to know your basic information, such as age, as well as your weight, height, gender, and general activity level. The macro calculator then calculates your individualized numbers.

For example, a 50-year-old woman who is moderately active and weighs 160 pounds at 5 feet, 4 inches, and wishes to lose weight will find that a macro calculator indicates she should consume no more than 1732 calories per day. She should distribute this caloric count as 74 percent (142 grams) fat, 21 percent (90 grams) protein, and six percent (25 grams) net carbs.

Useful Kitchen Tools

Making your keto meals from scratch is the most economical way to succeed on a keto diet, as processed foods will most likely contain ingredients on the no-go list. Opting out of packaged and prepared foods is ideal when embarking on keto. Therefore, it can help to have some particular kitchen gadgets at your disposal. A basic blender or even a smoothie maker is a handy tool not only for smoothie making but for mixing up your salad dressings and marinades.

Suppose you plan to substitute some carb-heavy foods like pasta with keto-friendly veggies (which we will dive into together in an upcoming chapter). In that case, you will want a 'zoodle maker,' sometimes called a spiralizer, which transforms zucchini, carrots, and other veggies into perfectly spiraled noodles you can use for any pasta dish.

A quality food processor tremendously helps when making your alternative rice dishes, such as cauliflower rice or broccoli rice.

While not necessary to purchase, if you already own a pressure cooker/slow cooker such as an Instapot or Ninja Foodi, these types of appliances can make perfect hard-boiled eggs, egg cups, and egg bites, as well as steam veggies. The slow cooker mode is ideal for planning your dinner well ahead of time. Remember, when you plan, you're more likely to stick to your keto meal plan and have success. If your pressure cooker appliance has an air fryer feature, this feature is ideal for preparing meat such as roasted chicken, fish, and steak.

It's not necessary to measure food portion sizes on a keto diet, but a food scale helps you weigh your food, so you can stay within your gram goals and limits, as explained above. Look for these features when you're ready to purchase a food scale for your kitchen.

- Conversion button: Most macro calculators and calorie-tracking apps allow you to toggle between US conversions and metric, but not all. It helps to have a conversion button on your scale to make the math easier.
- No automatic shut-off: An automatic shut-off feature can make measuring food more difficult. Find a scale that allows you to manually turn off this feature.
- Tare function: Most of the time, you'll want to measure your food in a container, bowl, or another vessel. What is called a tare function allows you to reset the weight at zero.
- Easy cleaning: Many scales have adopted a removable plate that is machine-washable, which can be extremely convenient when weighing messy foods.

And if you'll be eating a lot of avocado on your keto diet, and most do, you'll want an avocado keeper, which is a customized storage container that helps avocados last longer and keeps them from turning brown.

Keto Substitutions

I've discussed what you can and cannot eat on a keto diet, but for those items on the naughty list, what can you eat instead?

Hemp hearts instead of croutons on your salad: On a keto diet, every carb counts! Don't waste your daily allotment of 20-50 grams of net carbs on croutons. Instead, three tablespoons of hemp hearts contain only 1.4 grams of net carbs. You can find hemp hearts at most grocery stores and natural groceries.

Broccoli instead of green peas: Yes, I've said that most green vegetables are low in carbs, but the keyword is 'most.' Green peas are a starchy veggie, which means it contains more carbs than broccoli or even zucchini. Opt for one of these veggies, or fresh spinach, as a side to your meals instead of peas.

Sunflower seeds instead of 'low-fat' snacks: As we've already discussed together, low-fat or low-calorie do not equal low carb. Instead of snack packs of pretzels, granola, or chips, opt for sunflower seeds, which feel satisfying as a snack because they take longer to eat. Toasted pumpkin seeds and nuts are excellent alternatives.

Seaweed snacks instead of potato chips: Yes, you already know potato chips are on the restricted list, but what can you eat instead to satisfy that need for crispy, crunchy, salty goodness? Try packaged seaweed squares, which can be found in the snack aisle of your grocery store.

Berries instead of bananas: Bananas are healthy, but they're high in starch, and you already know that starch is a dangerous ingredient. Opt for a bowl of berries instead, perhaps topped with heavy cream if you want an extra dash of comfort food.

Deli meat instead of marinated meats: Check the labels, but many packaged deli meat are now keto-compliant. Opt for a turkey roll-up or ham slice with cheese in place of roasted ham with a glaze or meat marinated in honey or sugar-based rub.

EVOO instead of margarine: Extra virgin olive oil is a keto-friendly, fatty oil, so use it liberally in place of processed butter spreads. Remember, dairy butter is okay, but oils will be even better. Use EVOO on your salads, veggies, and meats during your keto diet.

Light beer instead of carb-heavy beer: Recheck your labels! Avoid most alcohol on a keto diet (most is pretty packed with carbs and sugar), but go ahead and enjoy an occasional light beer. Look for beers that pack less than six grams of carbs per can, if possible.

Cauliflower instead of sweet potatoes or russet potatoes: By now, you know what I'm going to say. Potatoes are packed with starches. Opt for riced cauliflower or cauliflower mash instead, which you can easily make in a food processor or even buy prepared in the frozen aisle of your local grocery store.

Almond milk or perhaps coconut milk instead of cow milk: You may have wondered why cream and butter are keto-friendly while cow's milk is not. This irregularity is because cow's milk has as much as 11 grams of carbs (in whole milk). If you put cow's milk in your smoothie, for instance, you may think you're staying keto-compliant, while in reality, you're drinking most of your allotment of carbs for the morning! Put almond milk in your smoothies instead. Just be sure to look for the unsweetened variety.

Salted nuts instead of trail mix: Many people consider trail mix a healthy snack option, but the sweetened, dried fruits and extras like chocolate chips or candied nuts can derail you quickly. Stick to nut mixes only, or snack on cheese cubes with your nuts.

Unsweetened sparkling water instead of soda: Skip the sugar and pick up a can of unsweetened, flavored seltzer water, such as La Croix. There are many brands and flavor varieties to choose from, which will help you not feel denied if you're a soda fan.

Spaghetti squash instead of a butternut squash: Most squashes are too starchy, just like potatoes.

But if you're craving something in the squash family, opt for spaghetti squash, which has the added benefit of mimicking noodles, too! You can make 'zoodles' out of zucchini, too, or any other veggie that suits you. Just remember that while carrots consumed in moderation are fine, they're not the best keto-friendly veggie, as they have more carbs, so make carrot zoodles sparingly.

Shirataki noodles instead of pasta: Zero calories noodles, or shirataki noodles, come from the root of a plant called the konjac. This plant grows in many parts of Asia. They are about 97 percent water and 3 percent glucomannan, which is a keto-friendly fiber. Shirataki noodles are a great choice because they are very filling. Use them in keto stir-fries or as a keto side dish to your meal. You'll feel like you are getting the carbs that you crave while you're actually avoiding them!

Coconut, egg, or cheese wraps instead of tortillas or sandwich bread: You can find packaged coconut wraps in your local natural foods store or online or make egg or cheese wraps yourself. Bake slices of cheese in the oven to create lightly crispy wraps (see my recipe in Chapter 7), or you can make egg crepes that have the same texture as tortillas.

Keto on a Budget

A keto diet is a perfect lifestyle choice if you don't have extra cash to spend inexpensive grocery store because it naturally relies on using whole foods and ingredients. You will save money every time you skip packaged and processed foods and every time you decide to skip dining out.

You will see keto-specific bars and snacks advertised to you, but you don't need to buy those if you don't want to! Processed foods are pricy, and keto snacks are even more expensive than most. Plus, they rarely taste excellent. Opt for snacks from our meal plan and recipes instead.

Meat is often a big part of a keto diet, and yes, meat can be expensive to purchase. Choose your cuts of meat carefully, however, and you can stay within a very reasonable budget. If you want beef, skip the rib eye and go for the roast cut. If you wish to pork, skip the bone-in and opt for the shoulder roast. Chicken thighs are usually cheaper than chicken breast. Utilize the knowledge of your local butcher or deli counter personnel, who can point you in the direction of prime cuts that cost less.

Shop at Trader Joe's or Grocery Outlet for whole foods and keto-friendly snack foods for a lower cost. These stores often feature bargains on healthy snack items, plus have many whole foods options, such as a robust produce and meat section at Trader Joe's.

Many budget grocery shoppers rely on buying canned beans to stretch their budget, but many beans are high in carbs, making them a less than great keto option. Skip black beans, which have as many as 11 net carbs per serving, and opt for soybeans if you need to supplement your grocery list with a lower-cost option.

Go ahead and eat plenty of berries on a keto diet, but keep in mind that they are sometimes the most expensive fruit in the store, depending on where you live and the season. Opt for frozen berries, which you can add to your meals for an icy, refreshing crunch in the warmer months, or which you can thaw or add to your smoothies year-round.

Join a farm share or a meat share to get local meat and local produce at a reasonable price. Sometimes better yet, get into the routine of patronizing your local farmer's market, which offers a plethora of fresh green, leafy vegetables, local meat cuts, and farm-fresh eggs.

Speaking of eggs, focus heavily on this food to stretch your budget further. Almost every keto meal that calls for meat can have eggs substituted instead, and this cheap food packs tons of protein.

I talked about how much it helps plan your keto meals for optimal success and less temptation to cheat, but planning your meals also enables you to save money. Use one cut of meat to create several keto dinners, or plan on leftovers for the next day's lunch. The more meals you have planned and prepared in your fridge, the less food waste you're likely to have.

Buy more expensive keto foods in bulk. Nuts, avocados, almond milk, and EVOO can be costly. Look for these items in bulk at stores like Grocery Outlet or Costco to save money in the long run. Costco is an excellent choice for meat jerky as well, as long as you read the ingredient list carefully to avoid sugar.

Supplements

Some people on a keto diet decide to add supplements. Because the keto diet eliminates many foods you might normally eat, it's essential to make sure you're still getting all the necessary nutrients. Some of these supplements can also help protect you against the adverse side effects of a keto diet, like the 'keto flu' I discussed earlier.

As with all dietary supplement use, consult your physician before adding over-the-counter supplements to your daily routine. Below are the most common supplements you may wish to add to your diet:

Magnesium: Magnesium boosts energy and helps regulate blood sugar. Due to a heavier reliance on processed foods, most people are deficient in magnesium. A keto diet is a great way to naturally up your magnesium intake, as you will be less reliant on processed foods as you prepare more fresh ingredients. Foods such as spinach, avocado, pumpkin seeds, kale, chard, and some fish, such as mackerel, are naturally high in magnesium.

Take 200-400 milligrams of magnesium a day to boost immunity and energy and relieve issues like muscle cramps or difficulty sleeping.

MCT oil: MCT, or medium-chain triglycerides, are ground down in the liver and before entering the bloodstream. Coconut oil is the best way to introduce MCT oil to your keto diet. Coconut oil will increase your fat intake, which in turn helps you achieve ketosis more efficiently. If you're already in ketosis, this oil can help you stay in ketosis longer.

MCT also helps with feelings of fullness, which can help you with your portion control while on your keto diet. Add coconut oil to your shakes or smoothies, use it for cooking oil, or even eat it by one spoonful a day!

Omega-3 fatty acids: When you picture omega-3s, you probably think of fish. This is because omega-3 fatty acids are located in fish oil. It contains eicosapentaenoic acid (EPA) and docosahexaenoic acid (DHA), which help reduce inflammation and lower heart risks. Don't confuse omega-3s with omega-6, which are fatty acids mostly hiding in processed foods and oil such as vegetable oil.

You can find omega-3 supplements at any health foods store or in the supplemental aisle of your local grocery store. Good and reliable brands provide a combined 500-600 milligrams of EPA and DHA per 1000 milligram per serving. If you are on blood-thinning medication, however, talk to your doctor before supplementing with omega-3s. If you prefer to supplement naturally, add more salmon, sardines, and anchovies to your keto diet.

Exogenous ketones: Your body naturally produces *endogenous* ketones through ketosis, whereas *exogenous* ketones must come from an external source. Exogenous ketones will help increase blood ketone levels. This increase can help you reach ketosis quicker, but it also aids with muscle recovery and decreased appetite. Buy ketone salts in an over-the-counter variety at most health food stores.

Greens powder: You already know you need to increase your intake of leafy green vegetables (who among us doesn't?). However, you can supplement your intake if you have trouble getting enough of these green vegetables into your keto diet naturally. Because keto focuses heavily on proteins, many keto dieters find themselves lacking in green vegetables.

Greens powder can be found at grocery stores and health food stores and usually contains a mixture of spinach, kale, broccoli, wheatgrass, and more. You can add greens powder to your smoothies and drinks. Just make sure you don't replace all your vegetable intake with a greens powder. One good way to consume your greens is by incorporating as many leafy green vegetables into your meals as possible.

Vitamin D: Everyone needs vitamin D, and vitamin D deficiencies are prevalent. Vitamin D is essential to your immune system and cell regrowth, and it promotes bone health by aiding in the absorption of calcium. Not many foods are decent sources of vitamin D, which is why many people choose a supplement.

Digestive enzymes: In the beginning days of a keto diet, the body is sometimes not used to the higher protein and fat intake. Digestive issues are fairly common as a result. For those who experience uncomfortable digestive problems like nausea, bloating, or diarrhea, adding a digestive enzyme supplement can help. These enzymes help you break down protein and help with muscle soreness, which is a plus for athletes.

Electrolytes: Ward against water loss in the body as you adapt to consuming fewer carbs. During the beginning days of a keto diet, sodium, potassium, and magnesium levels can sink, leading to headaches or fatigue. While a common side effect when a person first starts keto, electrolytes can alleviate this discomfort.

You can use electrolyte supplements to increase your sodium naturally by salting your food and eating plenty of nuts, avocados, and seeds.

Do you like what you're learning? Leave us an Amazon review! Reviews help others identify the most helpful keto guides available and allow me to continue doing what I love to do, empowering other women over 50 to find success!

Chapter 5: Tips for Keto Success

Many people have success on a keto diet because keto is relatively simple. There are not a lot of nutrition rules to follow, you don't have to constantly measure your food, and you can have the portions you need. Keto-friendly foods are naturally filling, and few people report feeling denied or cheated of their favorite indulgences while on keto.

This said, we all need all the help we can get, right? We can learn from those who have maintained a keto diet long-term, as well as those who are just starting along with us. It can be helpful to find accountability for your keto diet among family members or friends. Another source of inspiration and accountability is the internet. Find a keto success group or a keto diet Facebook group to join and be among people with similar success stories and challenges.

Tips for Entering Ketosis

After planning your keto meals and shopping for your keto-friendly foods, your first challenge will be entering ketosis (and staying there!). I have discussed how many women find success by gradually reducing their daily net carbs, shocking the body. Therefore, you may start out with as many as 70 net carbs per day, gradually reducing until you're at 20-50 net carbs. You may find it takes a bit longer to enter ketosis by taking this gradual approach, but your body will thank you.

As your body switches its primary main fuel source from glucose (sugar) to ketones, fat is broken down. This fact is great news for women who have a goal of losing weight on a keto diet. But how long can women over 50 expect ketosis to take?

As you drastically reduce your carbohydrate intake, your body will start dramatically using up its glycogen stores. But you can expect it to take 2-5 days to enter ketosis (and this is after you've reduced your carbs to the ideal 20-50 net carbs per day). Some people may find it takes as long as a week.

Why the variation in periods? Because it depends on your reliance on carbs before starting a keto diet. If you ate a high number of carbs in your previous daily diet, it would take your body longer to burn through its glycogen stores than if you ate a moderate amount of carbs. Either way, you're on your way to better health on a low-carb diet!

We've already learned how to tell when you're in ketosis, with symptoms that can include fatigue, nausea, and thirst. I also outlined tools you can use to help with your success, such as urine testing strips that measure ketone levels. You don't need to go out and buy an expensive blood ketone meter. You can simply tell whether you're in ketosis by looking for symptoms.

Common Mistakes That Delay Entering Ketosis

While you should have patience while waiting for your body to enter ketosis and remember that the process can take as long as one week, some people make some mistakes that can impede the process. These mistakes can include:

Eating more carbs than you think you're eating: You may think you're eating 50 net carbs a day, when in fact, you're consuming 90-100. How does this occur? Carbs can be sneaky! While you're getting used to a keto diet, you may need to scrutinize ingredient lists and nutritional guidelines more than you'd like.

Not eating enough fat: Most of us have had it beaten into us that fat is bad. We avoid eating high-fat foods. But on a keto diet, remember that heart-healthy fats are our friends. You should aim for 65-90 % of your daily calories to come from fat,

10-30 % from protein, and less than five % from carbs.

Eating too much protein: Reaching for more protein than fat while getting used to your keto diet is an easy mistake to make. But eating too much protein can make it harder to enter ketosis because protein consumption encourages your body to use gluconeogenesis, which is a process that converts amino acids from protein to sugar. And too much sugar stops your body from entering ketosis. Therefore, while you do have a green light to eat lots of protein on a keto diet, be sure to stay within the percentages recommended.

Not enough exercise: Want to get a head start on your ketosis process? Exercise more! Your body will burn through its carbs faster, helping you enter ketosis sooner. It's also important to get plenty of sleep and to try to avoid undue stress. What do we all do when we're stressed? We reach for the carbs!

Not tracking carbs: No one wants to track every calorie consumed, and on a keto diet, you don't have to! But while you get used to the nuances of your keto diet, you do need to track your net carbs. How else will you know if you're eating more than you think you are?

Using Intermittent Fasting to Boost Entering Ketosis

Many keto dieters report that intermittent fasting can help kick-start ketosis. Intermittent fasting is a method of consuming meals in which you cycle between periods of food consumption and periods of fasting. It's not a diet but rather a method of eating. Many people on a keto diet find the intermittent fasting method of eating to aid ketosis.

To use intermittent fasting on your keto diet, you first need to decide what percentage of time you'll spend fasting and what percentage you'll spending eating within a 24-hour period. Different fasting to eating ratios exist for different people.

Most people adopt a 16/8 ratio of intermittent fasting, which means that in a 24-hour period, they abstain from eating for 16 hours and eat during the remaining 8. For example, if you skip breakfast and eat your last meal of the day before 7 pm, you can break your fast and eat lunch at 11 am the next day.

The 5:2 method is another option. In this approach, you normally eat for five days of the week (on a keto diet) and then limit yourself to 500-600 calories only during two non-consecutive days of the week. This method can be challenging, but not as challenging as the 24-hour method, in which you fast for an entire 24 hour period during two non-consecutive days a week.

For most women over age 50, a modified 16/8 ratio can be best. For example, many women over 50 prefer a 12/10 ratio. This type is the most straightforward form of intermittent fasting to stick to because you only have to remember to skip breakfast daily.

Why does fasting help? Obviously, fasting ensures you consume fewer calories overall (provided that you don't compensate by eating too many calories later in the day).

Also, when you fast, your body's hormones make stored fat more accessible. The faster we burn through that stored fat, the quicker we're in ketosis. Fasting has many additional benefits as well, including the increase of your Human Growth Hormone (HGH) by as much as five-fold. This increase also helps burn fat and build muscle.

Intermittent fasting also aids in cellular repair and improves insulin sensitivity, allowing insulin levels to drop. Gene expression changes also occur, helping the body with long-term disease prevention.

When you add intermittent fasting to your keto diet, you can often boost ketosis while gaining many other health benefits in the process.

Tips for Long-Term Keto Diet Success

Once you've entered ketosis, now what? It's time to focus on staying there! Your keto meal plans are your best tool for keto success because when we know what we're eating and have a plan, we curb unintentional snacking and avoid moments when keto-friendly foods are not available to us. In addition to keto meal planning, adapt the following keto success tips:

Eliminate processed foods: Not all processed foods are on the keto diet no-no list, but most are! To simplify your keto diet, try to simply avoid all processed foods. If you have to rip open a package or box to eat it, it's processed and probably not keto-friendly food. Plus, processed foods are calorie-dense ad usually filled with sugar as well.

Stay away from sugar substitutes: You know not to eat sugar, but what about those natural sweeteners, like honey and maple syrup? No, and no. The same goes for agave. For a sweet taste, opt for coconut oil. You can even make 'bulletproof coffee' by adding a dollop of coconut oil to your morning cup of joe.

Change your attitude about food: Do you use food as a reward? As a comfort on bad days? We all do, sometimes. There's a reason why movies so often depict a crying woman eating a tub of ice cream after a breakup, after all. But we can choose to change our relationship with food. When you adopt a keto diet, you start to view food as a fuel source, not a reward or a comfort.

Start simple: Even with a meal plan in place, starting keto can feel intimidating. Start simple with some of your favorite foods or most familiar foods. This formula can help with any meal:

- Pick a protein: chicken, beef, pork, fish, eggs, sugar-free nut butter, or protein powder
- Pick a veggie: cauliflower, broccoli, Brussel sprouts, or any other low-carb veggie
- Pick a fat: butter, oil, lard, ghee, cheese, cream, bacon, avocado, mayonnaise, nuts

Remove temptations: This tip can be tough to follow if you live with others who are not on a keto diet. However, it's still possible to keep tempting foods out of sight and out of mind. Designate a drawer or cupboard for your keto-friendly snacks and ingredients and avoid the need to open any other kitchen storage areas. And of course, if everyone in your household is on board with a keto diet, rid the entire house of packaged, processed foods that contain too many carbs and sugars.

Plan to grocery shop more often: You will be purchasing more fresh vegetables, which means your dinner and lunch ingredients may spoil faster than you're used to (especially if you often rely on processed foods that contain more preservatives). But grocery shopping for keto ingredients can be part of the fun of a keto diet, and the deliberate act of thinking through your meals and planning your recipes can help you stay on track.

Find online support: Trust us; your friends and family who are not subscribing to a keto diet will get tired of hearing you talk about it! But it's important to get encouragement and help from others. Online support groups, keto challenge groups, and help forums can be a great place to get the community you might need.

Don't weigh or measure yourself too often: It's very easy to get discouraged if you weigh yourself daily on a keto diet. Instead, keep yourself accountable with a weigh-in about one time per week, at the same time each week. Keto results will vary, but as long as you're losing a couple of pounds per week, you're doing well (assuming weight loss is your goal). Some women also find themselves hitting a plateau after initial success. If this happens to you, try a week of intermittent fasting or recalculate your macros.

Prioritize sleep and avoid stress: Yes, we all would like to do both of these things all of the time, but while on a keto diet, it's more important than ever to get enough rest and feel relaxed. Tired and stressed out people overeat, cheat on their diet, and feel discouraged or negative. It doesn't seem like sleeping a lot would help a person lose weight, but it does!

Make sure you're getting enough salt: Try bone broth or Himalayan sea salt containing trace minerals. Consuming plenty of salt can help you avoid an electrolyte imbalance, which is when your electrolytes decrease with your decrease in carbs, causing unwanted side effects such as leg or muscle cramps, constipation, headaches, and shakiness or dizziness.

Exercise often: The more you exercise, the faster your body burns through its glycogen stores. And remember, once this happens, it looks for other sources of fuel. It will turn to fat for energy, which will help you become leaner and lose weight. Be sure to incorporate high-intensity activities with low-intensity activities for the best results. Look for more exercise tips in a later chapter.

Batch cook: By cooking up most of your week's meals at once, you not only save time but you more readily ensure that you will eat all your keto-friendly meals. You won't want those ingredients, which are already cooked and ready to go, to go to waste. Batch cooking helps you feel more prepared for your day's keto structure and allows you to resist the temptation to reach for non-friendly snack food.

Drink lots of water: Drinking the eight glasses always recommended by experts per day makes you feel fuller and keep you hydrated no matter what diet you are following. On a keto diet, you will excrete more water because you are consuming fewer carbs. An easy rule of thumb to remember: aim to drink at least half of your actual body weight in oz of water per day. Yes, this sounds like too much, but it isn't!

Ensure you have strong gut health: Gut health is a big topic these days. When your body's gut flora is healthy, your hormones, insulin sensitivity, and metabolism follow suit. To improve your gut health, drink plenty of water (yes, this again!). You will also want to ensure you get enough sleep, eat slowly during meals, and consider taking a prebiotic and probiotic supplement.

Success When Dining Out on Keto

Yes, you can experience success on a keto diet while dining out at restaurants. It will be easier to stick to your keto diet if you don't dine out too often, but life happens, and sometimes we find ourselves dining out. We don't want to avoid life or avoid spending time with family and friends, so keep the following tips in mind when at a restaurant.

Be aware of some pitfalls of dining out. First of all, most restaurants offer too-large portion sizes, so it can help to begin your meal by asking for a to-go box and boxing a portion of your meal before you even start.

Beware of added sugars and carbs hiding in plain sight. Beware of dressings, sauces, and breading on proteins (such as breaded chicken or fried fish).

You have already learned that you can calculate net carbs by taking the total carbs and subtracting the grams of fiber and sugar. This fact is because net carbs are what wreak havoc on your blood sugar level and compromise weight loss. But neither the government nor the Academy of Nutrition and Dietetics recognizes the net carbs term, so you won't find this information readily available on nutritional information on menus. You'll have to do the hard work of the calculations yourself.

The best way to go about finding a keto-friendly meal at a restaurant is to start with a slice of simply-prepared meat, such as grilled chicken, then adding sides a la carte, such as a green vegetable and a salad. Cheese is a good option but beware of prepared cheese sauces that might be hiding sugar.

Don't be afraid to ask about substitutions, such as cauliflower rice in place of rice pilaf or an extra serving of vegetables in place of a baked potato. Many restaurants now offer a substitution of a lettuce wrap in place of a bun, too.

The good news is, a keto diet is becoming more common, and most restaurants now recognize and understand such requests. And the more people request keto-friendly foods, and the more restaurants will provide them!

Look for Keto-Friendly Foods on the Menu

At breakfast, you can almost always find bacon and eggs on a menu. Go this route! If the menu indicates that your eggs come with pancakes or toast, substitute for more eggs or another breakfast meat.

At lunch, it's easy to find salad choices. Ask for the salad dressing to be replaced with oil and vinegar. Top your salad with grilled chicken or diced hard-boiled eggs, or opt for a tuna salad with mayonnaise.

Dinners at restaurants often feature a signature cut of meat as a main dish, so it's easy to opt for a steak, a filet of salmon or halibut, or grilled chicken. Replace sides of potatoes or rolls with extra servings of low-carb vegetables, and don't shy away from adding on extra butter, salt, or sour cream.

Charcuterie plates with cured meats (just make sure they don't have added sugar), sliced cheeses, veggies, olives, and nuts are an excellent option if someone wants to share a plate for the table. Other keto-friendly appetizers include veggie sticks, salads, and stuffed mushroom caps (with sausage, cheese, or beef).

Pick a Keto-Friendly Restaurant

The following well-known restaurant chains have keto-friendly options on their menu.

Applebee's: The basic premise of Applebee's is to offer plenty of grilled meat options, making it ideal for those on a keto diet. Opt for lean meat with Applebee's fire-roasted vegetables on the side.

Chili's: Like Applebee's, Chili's best attribute is its simplicity. Get a classic steak with a side of broccoli or grilled veggie and chicken skewers. Remember to beware of hidden carbs and sugars in sauces and gravies.

Starbucks: Starbucks' grab-and-go section of most stores is full of keto-friendly options. Try their meat and cheese boxes, o tr nut butter, hard-boiled egg, and cheese breakfast trays in the prepared food cases. Another good pick is their egg bites (depending on the type.)

Olive Garden: Surprised? You shouldn't be! You don't have to order pasta at Olive Garden, and this chain offers grilled meat options, including their grilled salmon filet. Olive Garden's popular salad bowl with Italian dressing is an okay choice as well, as long as you remember that you'll be consuming 11 net carbs in the salad dressing (per serving). Antipasto salad is always a good pick, too.

International House of Pancakes: Yes, IHOP is known for its pancakes, but its build-your-own egg dish is the perfect keto meal! Add in plenty of green veggies, bacon, and cheeses (avocado and spinach are great veggie choices).

Cheesecake Factory: As long as you can step through the door and resist the temptation for cheesecake, the Cheesecake Factory has good keto options for you. Their pan-seared branzino is a delicious white fish served with lemon butter and veggies on the side.

TGI Fridays: Like Chili's and Applebee's, TGI Fridays has a wide variety of grilled meat dishes to choose from. Plus, they have some keto-friendly salads, such as their cobb with grilled chicken. You can add blue cheese, and even the Ranch dressing only has two net carbs per serving.

Outback Steakhouse: Get a lobster tail or grilled shrimp, as neither skimp on the garlic herb butter. A steak is a valid choice as well. You'll just have to skip the deep-fried blooming onion they're known for.

Red Lobster: Like Outback Steakhouse, Red Lobster has a plethora of seafood options to pick between. Their snow crab or their lobster tail are great picks. Yes, it won't be fun to skip their biscuits, but you will be happy you did during your next weigh-in.

California Pizza Kitchen: This chain is known for many healthy dining out options with many fresh ingredients. Try one of their many salads with a vinaigrette dressing.

Boston Market: Boston Market's rotisserie chicken is a fantastic keto choice, and you can pair it with a Caesar salad. Opt for the dark chicken meat, as it has more fat.

Red Robin: Their burgers can be made with lettuce wraps instead of buns. Opt for their guacamole bacon burger, which is packed with flavor but very low on carbs.

Denny's: Bacon and eggs, scrambles with cheese and veggies, and sausage is all excellent breakfast picks. And remember that Denny's makes dinner, too, with grilled chicken and fish options.

Buffalo Wild Wings: Chicken wings are an excellent keto food, as long as you're careful about the sweet sauces. Opt for a spicier sauce to reduce your carb load.

Keto-Friendly Fast Food

Au Bon Pain: Try the breakfast or lunch bar options, or get an egg, sausage, and cheese sandwich without the bagel.

Shack Shack: Get their burgers on a lettuce wrap, and you're good to go! You can also get a bunless chicken dog for more variety.

Baja Fresh: Build your own with a bed of lettuce, topped with chicken, guacamole, cheese, and Pico de Gallo.

KFC: Try their grilled chicken, and skip the high-carb sides in favor of green beans.

Arby's: Meat-centric Arby's is a good choice because of their loaded-up roast beef and brisket. And now, you can ask for it without the bun or bread and simply tackle your meat and cheese with a fork. The turkey farmhouse salad is also a good option.

Subway: Their double chicken chopped salad is a good pick, as are any of their salads since you can customize them to you. Ask for plenty of veggies and meats and cheeses, and top it all off with a low-carb Ranch or a vinaigrette dressing.

Del Taco: Mexican food is ripe with good keto options. At Del Taco, try their chicken bacon avocado salad (without the tortilla chips) or their Fresca bowl without the rice.

Freshii: Everything is customizable and fresh at Freshii, making it a perfect bet for those on a keto diet. Their green eggs and kale salads a good pick, as is the Mediterranean bowl and their salads.

Whataburger: Whataburger is a staple for some families, and their patty melt or grilled chicken salad is very keto-friendly, as is their bunless avocado bacon burger.

Restaurants With Dedicated Keto Meals or Menus

Chipotle: I love that Chipotle now has a keto salad or keto bowl option, both of which are bursting with meat, guacamole, cheeses, and salsa.

Jimmy John's: Their 'Unwich' is a sandwich served on a lettuce wrap instead of bread. A great pick is their tuna salad, made with mayonnaise. Their Cubano Unwich is also a great option.

Panera Bread: Their power breakfast bowl is a keto staple! You can choose between an egg white bowl with turkey or an egg bowl with steak. Both come with veggies mixed in.

Five Guys: I love that Five Guys lets you do a bunless bowl for any burger or hot dog combination. And there are so many toppings to add that are keto-friendly, such as pickles, onion, tomato, and more. They use almost all clean, whole foods, and the boiled peanuts that are always free are also keto-friendly!

Qdoba: This fast-food chain features a Smoked Brisket Keto Bowl as one of their Lifestyle Bowl options. You can also customize their taco salad with chicken to be keto-compliant.

In-N-Out: It's so easy to order a keto meal at In-N-Out! Ask for the protein double-double or any bunless hamburger of your choice. Sadly, you'll have to forgo the fries and the shakes, but you can top your burger with plenty of cheese!

Foods to Always Avoid While Dining Out

No matter where you dine out, always remember to skip the following while ordering:

- Anything fried
- Bread or buns of any sort
- Potatoes
- Most side dishes
- Sweet sauces or gravies (especially barbeque sauces)
- Creamy or thick soups
- Corn-based foods like croutons or cornmeal encrusted meats
- Desserts

Foods to Gravitate Toward

- Balsamic dressings
- Oil and vinegar
- Mayonnaise-based foods
- Simple cuts of meat
- Green leafy veggies
- Cheese
- Butter
- Eggs

Chapter 6: Getting Exercise While on a Keto Diet

Can you exercise while on a keto diet? Yes, but the answer is more complicated than just go for it. While many experts have attributed improved blood sugar and increased fat-burning to a keto diet, others worry the low-carb diet can lower energy levels in some people, especially those whose athletic performance is high. Extreme exercise can also challenge muscle growth.

However, if you're not an extreme athlete, it's a great idea to add exercise to your daily routine, along with your keto diet. A low-carb lifestyle works well with endurance sports, so whereas you might not feel an increase of short bursts of energy on keto, you will likely have more energy overall. Why is physical endurance increased while in ketosis? Because the body has become so much more efficient at burning fat for energy!

And if you've decided to take any of the supplements I recommended to stay in ketosis, these increased levels of ketones may speed muscle strength. Overall, more research is needed to know if a keto diet has long-lasting and substantial benefits for endurance, fat-burning, and muscle recovery. It's important that you remember: a keto diet largely consists of consuming fats, so naturally, you *burn* more fat on a keto diet. In other words, these two facts may equal each other out. But exercise has not been shown to impede a keto diet on a long-term basis. What does this mean for you? We all know how important exercise can be for staying fit and healthy, overall, no matter what diet you're following.

Some Symptoms to Expect on a Keto Diet That Impact Exercise

You may find that you feel less energy than usual when you are getting used to ketosis. Because you are severely decreasing your daily intake of carbs, which are your body's main source of energy, you will feel sluggish at first. This feeling can make exercise feel less appealing in the early days of your diet. Stick with it, however, because several studies have shown that while athletes on a keto diet reported decreased energy levels in the first week, their energy gradually improved until they reported their usual energy levels over time.

You will most likely experience weight loss on a keto diet, increasing feelings of fatigue as ketone levels rise. Short bouts of intense exercise may prove difficult on keto, which is why many women focus on more endurance-based exercise.

Tip: if you consider yourself an extreme athlete, are focused on building muscle, or plan to compete in an intense competition during the time you're on a keto diet, consult your physician before starting. A modified keto diet, with less restriction on carbs, may be right for you.

Even if you have to start out easy and gradually work up to a full exercise routine, any and all physical activity will be beneficial to your body. Remember, a sedentary lifestyle has been attributed to many chronic health issues that women over 50 are at risk for. The best way to avoid feeling unwell or chronically sick is to move your body every day. Always slowly start if you need to, and feel your body get leaner, toned, and stronger!

Best Exercises on a Keto Diet

So what exercise should you pursue while on a restricted carb diet? Low intensity, steady-state exercise is best. It's the short bursts of varied moves that will likely drain you. Therefore, interval training, such as the HIIT (high-intensity interval training) classes you often find in an Orange Theory cardio studio or a Peloton running course, is not your friend right now. High-intensity exercise is glycolytic, meaning it requires the burning of glucose as fuel. Once you're keto-adapted, you can use your glucose stores for fuel, so you can slowly reintroduce these high-intensity bursts of exercise as your body gets used to being in ketosis. But for now, focus on endurance running or rowing.

If your workout routine normally includes a lot of high-impact activities, work low-impact exercise gradually. Want to hang onto your high-intensity workouts? That may be a bad idea because of the way your body creates energy. High-intensity workouts use energy burned by sugar, of which you are in short supply when you are on ketosis. Low-intensity workouts use energy burned by fat, which is your goal.

The following are excellent keto diet exercise options:

Lifting Weights

Why? Strength training offers a better metabolic effect than most cardio workouts. Just make sure you're getting hot and sweaty and getting your heart rate up while you lift. Focus on dense, lean muscle mass. Ketosis is a great time to build lean muscle and focus on your strength! If you have a hard time getting any cardio benefits while lifting, it's okay to pair a weight training session with 20 minutes on the treadmill or stairclimber to pick up your heart rate.

Make sure to focus on a high-rep, low-weight routine when lifting weights at the start of keto. This type of resistance training best works with your body on ketosis. Think 'endurance' for weight training...lots of lifting of lighter weights. You may even wish to begin with a bodyweight option (lifting using only your body weight, such as a lunge or a squat).

Jogging

Maybe you can jog around the block while your child or grandchild rides a bike, or perhaps you can jog with your dog or a friend. Start out easy if jogging is new to your routine, planning to jog only one-third of the time, walking two-thirds of the time. Begin with a short distance or a time limit (20 minutes can be a good starting point). You can simply work your way up from there.

Biking

If jogging or running hurts your knees or other joints, biking can be an excellent alternative. Use a stationary bike, pair it with a fitness app such as Peloton or Nike, and follow the low-impact endurance ride options. (Be sure to avoid their HIIT rides for now.) If biking outside, find a rail trail or bike path near your home for the most relaxing way to exercise while cycling.

Rowing

A rowing machine is a staple for many women who love cardio classes, but you can do an endurance row without the high bursts of cardio activity. Alternatively, rent or buy a paddleboard or kayak and row on a calm body of water near your home when the weather permits.

Swimming is also an excellent low-impact cardio activity that is often easy on older adults' joints and knees. Swim at your local club or YMCA year-round, or opt for outdoor swims during the warmer months, depending on your climate.

Walking

Like running, biking, and jogging, walking is an extremely accessible exercise option. Just step outside your door and go! Take the kids, take the dogs, or grab a willing (or maybe a reluctant!) partner or friend, and make a plan to walk 30 minutes a day, every day.

Yoga

Yoga classes are more readily available than ever before, thanks to the number of streaming exercise services and apps today. Start with a beginning flow class, which will work through the whole body, toning muscle and focusing on balance and core strength. Hot yoga is a great option to get the heart rate up higher and work up a sweat, and meditative or relaxation yoga is a wonderful way to unwind at the end of a busy day.

Pilates, barre, and gymnastics are also excellent choices for exercise during keto that focus on balance and toning, just like yoga. No one needs to join a costly gym to try these types of classes. Check out the many free versions on YouTube or other sources online to try before you buy. When you find a type of class you love, only then might it be a good investment to purchase a membership on an app, buy a piece of exercise equipment, or head to a physical gym to work out.

Tip: Remember, you don't have to avoid cardio exercise on a keto diet! You just need to make sure you're aiming for low-impact cardio instead of HIIT. Cardio is a great way to build endurance. Don't shy away from exercise while on a keto diet. Listen to how your body feels and allow for rest days, but also trust that your wants want to move, and with the right fuel, can perform better than you might even imagine when you're consuming keto-friendly foods.

Seven-Day Exercise Routine for Keto Dieters

Day 1: Bodyweight resistance training:
Three sets each of:
- 15 squats
- 15 reverse lunges
- 15 glute ham raises (raising on tip-toe)

20 minutes low-impact cardio of your choice (running, jogging, walking, swimming, rowing)

Day 2:
Bodyweight training:
- 10 push-ups (on knees if needed)
- 20 sit-ups or crunches
- 20 sit-up twists (right elbow to left knee, and the reverse)

20 minutes low-impact walking

Day 3:
Weight training:
Three sets each of:
- 15 deadlifts (heavy weights)
- 15 glute bridges
- 15 low rows (light weights)

30 minutes of Pilates or yoga

Day 4:
Bodyweight training:
Three sets each of:

- 30-second plank 30-second squats
- 15 bicycle rows

20 minutes low-impact cardio of your choice

Day 5:
Weight training:
Three sets each of:
- 15 bicep curls
- 15 overhead presses
- 15 bent-over rows

30 minutes yoga, barre, or Pilates

Day 6:
REST DAY

Day 7:
Bodyweight training:
Body weight for each of:
- 10 burpees
- 10 lunge jumps
- 50 jumping jacks

20 minutes biking or jogging

Tip: If you have any restrictions, such as weak wrists or ankles, an injured knee, or arthritic joints, you can find modifications. For example, hold a plank on your elbows instead of push-ups if your wrists hurt when holding body weight. Try static lunges instead of hopping lunges if you have issues with your knees.

Tips for Keto Exercise Success

To be successful, remember that if you mess up and fail to exercise one day, you should not beat yourself up about it. Just get right back to it the next day! Enlist an exercise buddy or at least be self-accountable by posting your exercise plan where others can see it (and encourage you!) in your home.

Plan your meals so you're never hungry when you're ready to exercise, and make sure you continue to get enough calories. You can't have a balanced, successful exercise plan without enough calories to fuel it. Remember that on a low-carb diet, energy breakdown is slower than on a high-carb diet. It's normal to feel a bit sluggish at times, which is why you're kind to yourself, focusing on low-impact exercise.

Stick to a daily routine, exercising at the same time each day. It can help to dress for success because when you get up and put your exercise clothing on, you're far more likely to follow through with your exercise plan! It's also important to get enough sleep each night and to drink enough water. Always drink 8-10 cups of water a day, if not more, while on a keto diet.

How to Fuel Your Keto Exercise

There's a lot to remember while on a keto diet, but try to keep in mind that at its core, food is fuel. When you exercise, you need to make sure you are properly fueling your body. As we discussed, your keto diet, and being in ketosis, is likely new to your body. You will feel fatigued. As your body makes adjustments and learns to burn fat in new ways, you need to be extra kind to yourself and pay close attention to your body's needs.

If your primary goal on your keto diet (and in your keto exercise routine) is to lose some weight, you'll want to keep your carb consumption as low as possible, of course, but you may also want to watch your fat intake more than is customary on keto. Slowly but steadily lower your fat intake until you have reduced 500 calories a day in this category.

If your primary goal is muscle gain or improved athletic performance in your sport, you will want to increase your fat consumption while exercising on a keto diet. You'll want to add about 300-500 calories per day in fat intake (not in carbs). You will also want to increase your protein intake when on keto.

If your primary goal is endurance for sports like road running or cycling, you will want to follow guidance for fat intake as 70 percent of macros. You will probably start at the highest allotment of carbs (around 50 grams per day), but you will gradually increase this once you're in ketosis. As described earlier, you will also want to utilize the supplements available to you, such as MCT oils, to fuel your endurance workouts.

When to Decrease or Stop exercise While on a Keto Diet

While daily low-impact exercise is a great idea for most people on a keto diet, it's essential to listen to your body and know when you may need to slow down or adjust your workout routine. Some women over age 50 will find that they are more successful when they focus solely on the nutritional aspects of a keto diet and forego exercise until they feel more energy returning. This option is especially true for women who feel the keto flu more intensely. Push through this period, however, and you will feel your energy returning and be able to work out again.

Additional reasons for decreasing or stopping daily exercise while in ketosis include:

Suppose your primary care provider restricts your exercise due to a health concern or injury. If this is the case, ask about the benefits of a keto diet before embarking upon a keto journey. And stick with the limited exercise or movement you were previously prescribed. You can still lose weight on a keto diet without adding exercise to your daily routine. You will simply have to be stricter about your net carbs.

Suppose you have had a hip or knee replacement. You don't need to stop exercise, but you will need to consult with your doctor and stick to prescribed movements. You can also find alternatives to standard exercises by listing restrictions in whatever exercise app or program you are using.

Suppose you are battling keto flu. Take a break from exercise, as described above. Make sure you are drinking plenty of water (at least eight glasses per day) and getting plenty of sleep. This period will pass. Perhaps try to take one short daily walk during this time.

The good news is, almost everyone can participate in low-impact cardio. After all, we all do at least one low-impact cardio 'exercise' every day: walking! If a full exercise routine intimidates you, plan on walking every day. One idea: take the stairs at work or school instead of the elevator, park further away in the parking lot than necessary or walk to get the mail or the paper. Make a plan to walk!

Chapter 7: Keto Recipes

I've already outlined why it's a great idea to plan on a keto diet for optimal success. Part of planning involves keeping your keto meal log current (which you'll have an opportunity to download in the next section) and creating a keto meal plan for each week. Keto recipes are intuitive and easy—remember, at its core, a keto meal is simply a protein, a veggie, and a portion of fats—and most likely, many of the recipes you already use on a weekly or monthly basis are keto-friendly. And many more are easily adapted to be keto-compliant.

Replace mashed potatoes in your favorite dish for cauliflower mash, for instance, or replace pasta with zoodles. Most of your meat dishes will already be compliant, as long as you keep a careful eye on the ingredient list to ward off sneaky sugars and carbs. It will be easier to stay away from kinds of pasta, grains, starches, and bread than you might think, especially with some ready-to-go recipes at your disposal.

Below, you'll find a sampling of top keto-friendly recipes to aid in your planning. Consider these meals to be an inspiration and a launching point for you to get more creative. Almost all the meats and veggies in these meals can be substituted with others based on your family's personal preferences, and some recipes may remind you of meals you already make and love. Feel free to adjust and adapt these recipes to your preferences, bearing in mind keto-compliant and non-compliant foods. You'll have the opportunity to download a master list of keto-compliant foods and restricted foods in the next section, which you can keep handy for easy reference. You can also refer to the substitutions I outlined in Chapter 5 if you get stuck!

Ready to plan some keto-friendly meals? Below, you will find options for breakfast, lunch, and dinner. Refer to the many keto snack ideas outlined in the keto meal planning section if you need different ideas between meals. However, these keto breakfasts and lunch ideas fill, which means you'll find less temptation to snack! Let's get started.

Keto Breakfast Recipes

Keto-Style Nutty Granola

Total Prep & Cooking Time: 45 min.
Yields: 3 Cups

Ingredients:

- Cooking spray
- 1 c. walnuts
- 1 c. almonds
- 1 c. coconut flakes - unsweetened
- ¼ c. sesame seeds
- 2 tbsp. chia seeds, whole
- 2 tbsp. flaxseeds
- 1 t. ground cinnamon
- 1 egg white
- 1 t. vanilla extract
- ¼ c. melted coconut oil

Set the oven temperature to reach 350 degrees. Lightly grease a baking tray. Chop the nuts. Mix the almonds, walnuts, coconut flakes, and seeds. Stir in spices and extract. Beat egg white, then stir this mixture into the granola along with the coconut oil.

Pour mixture onto the sheet in one even layer and bake for 20-25 minutes. Let cool completely before eating with almond milk for a keto cereal option, or snack on this granola plain or over a bed of berries.

Sausage and Egg Sandwich

Total Prep & Cooking Time: 20 min.
Yields: 3 Servings

Ingredients:

- 6 large eggs
- 2 tbsp. heavy cream
- Pinch of black pepper and salt
- Pinch of red pepper flakes
- 1 tbsp. butter
- 3 slices cheddar cheese
- 6 frozen sausage patties, heated through
- Sliced avocado if preferred

Whisk the eggs with the cream, salt, pepper flakes, and black pepper in a mixing container. Melt butter using a med-high temperature setting. Scoop the first third of the egg mixture into the skillet and cook until done to your preference. Top with one slice of cheddar cheese and allow to melt. Remove from pan and plate the dish - continue using the rest of the egg mixture until you have three egg portions completed. Serve the eggs between two sausage patties with sliced avocado in the middle to form an egg and sausage sandwich.

Keto-Friendly Pancakes

Total Prep & Cooking Time: 20 min.
Yields: 10 Servings

Ingredients:

- ½ cup almond flour
- 4 eggs
- 4 oz. unchilled cream cheese
- Butter, for frying and serving
- Pinch of cinnamon, if preferred

Using a bowl, go ahead and whisk together the almond flour, eggs, cream cheese, and cinnamon until smooth. Melt at least one tablespoon of butter in a non-stick skillet using a medium-temperature setting. Pour in approximately three tablespoons of batter. Cook until golden brown, flip, and transfer to a serving plate. Continue this process until all batter is cooked. Serve with butter and top with additional cinnamon if preferred.

Keto Berry-Delicious Smoothie

Total Prep & Cook Time: 5 min.
Yields: 4 Portions

Ingredients:

- 1 ½ c. frozen raspberries
- 1 ½ cup frozen strawberries
- 1 ½ c. frozen blackberries
- 1 c. spinach, chopped
- 2 c. almond or coconut milk

Blend all ingredients until they are creamy smooth. Pour into chilled mugs. Garnish using a portion of coconut flakes or more berries if preferred.

Breakfast Egg and Veggie Cups

Total Prep & Cooking Time: 25 min.

Yields: 6 Servings

Ingredients:

- 12 eggs
- 2 tbsp. chopped onion
- ¼ c. shredded cheddar

Optional additions

- ¼ cup chopped spinach
- ¼ c. chopped bacon
- ¼ c. chopped red bell pepper
- ¼ c. sliced mushrooms
- ¼ tsp. garlic powder
- ¼ c. grape or cherry tomatoes, chopped

Preheat 350 degrees. Lightly spray a muffin tin (coconut oil is best). In the bowl of your choice, whisk together eggs, onion, and cheddar cheese (or any cheese of your choice). Fold in any additional ingredients. Pour mixture into muffin tins, filling ¾ to the top. Set a timer to bake them for 15 or 20 minutes. Cool before serving. This dish can also be refrigerated for up to three days.

Keto Chocolate Protein Shake

Total Prep & Cooking Time: 5 min.
Yields: 1 Serving

Ingredients:

- ½ c. collagen powder
- ¼ c. powdered Erythritol
- 2 tbsp. flax meal
- ¼ cup cacao powder or unsweetened cocoa powder

Optional add-ins

- Egg white protein powder
- Almond butter
- Coconut milk powder
- Ground chia seeds

Blend all ingredients until smooth. Serve in a chilled glass.

Keto Breakfast Sausage Roll-Ups

Total Prep & Cooking Time: 15 min.
Yields: 5 Servings

Ingredients:

- 10 eggs, lightly beaten
- ½ pound ground sausage
- 10 slices mozzarella cheese
- Pinch of salt

Set the oven temperature to reach 400 degrees.
Cook sausage through and add the eggs. Cook until
scrambled, then set aside. Line a sheet of your
choice with parchment paper and lay mozzarella
slices on top. Bake until the cheese starts to brown
(5-6 min.). Transfer the pan to the countertop to
cool. Divide the sausage and egg mixture among the
cheese slices, rolling the cheese around the mixture
like a burrito.

Add-ins for this recipe can include jalapenos, red
bell pepper, mushroom, bacon, broccoli, onion, or
any other keto-friendly food!

Cured Salmon and Eggs

Total Prep & Cooking Time: 10 min.
Yields: 4 Servings

Ingredients:

- 8 slices cured salmon (or smoked salmon if preferred)
- 8 eggs, lightly beaten
- ½ c. shredded cheese of your choice if preferred
- ¼ c. diced green onion
- ¼ c. sour cream
- 1 avocado, sliced
- Pinch of salt

In a non-stick skillet, scramble eggs, adding in cheese if using. Once done, transfer to plates and top with diced green onion and a dollop of sour cream. Add cured salmon to each plate and garnish with sliced avocado.

Avocado and Bacon Deviled Eggs

Total Prep & Cooking Time: 35 min.
Yields: 4 Servings

Ingredients:

- 6 eggs
- 3-4 bacon slices
- ¼ c. mayonnaise
- 1 avocado
- 1 tsp. yellow mustard (unsweetened)
- 1 tsp. white vinegar
- Pinch of black pepper and salt

Follow your preferred method for hard-boiling eggs. Meanwhile, cook the bacon per the package directions in a non-stick skillet, allow to cool, and chop.

Peel eggs and slice them lengthwise, removing yolks into a large bowl. Reserve the egg whites as your cups for your deviled eggs. Mash the yolks first, then add the remaining ingredients, except bacon. Scoop the yolk mixture into your egg white cups and top with crumbled bacon.

Keto lunch recipes

BLTA Keto-Friendly Lettuce Wraps

Total Prep & Cooking Time: 10 min.
Yields: 4 Servings

Ingredients:

- •8 slices bacon, cooked
- •4 large lettuce leaves, for wrap
- •1 large tomato, sliced
- •2 large avocados, sliced
- •Pinch of salt

Wash and dry lettuce leaves, and open on a clean work surface. Evenly distribute sliced tomato, sliced avocado, and sliced bacon between the leaves, top with salt, and roll.

Creamy Chicken Cobb Salad

Total Prep & Cook Time: 15-16 min.
Yields: 4 Servings

Ingredients:

- 4 hard boiled eggs
- 12 oz. chopped chicken breast, cooked
- 2 avocados, diced
- 8 bacon slices, chopped
- Pinch of pepper and salt
- 1 small red onion, chopped
- 1/3 c. mayonnaise
- 1 ½ tbsp. lemon juice
- 1/3 c. sour cream
- 2 tbsp. chopped fresh dill
- 2 tsp. Dijon mustard
- Romaine lettuce, chopped

Toss the chicken, bacon, onion, avocados, and hard-boiled eggs. Stir together the mayo, sour cream, dill, lemon juice, mustard, salt, pepper, and fold into the salad mixture. Distribute chopped lettuce between bowls and top with the Cobb mixture.

Zesty Sesame Chicken

Total Prep & Cook Time: 25 min.
Yields: 4 Servings

Ingredients:

- ¼ c. soy sauce or coconut aminos
- 1 tbsp. rice vinegar
- ¼ c. unsweetened ketchup
- 1 tbsp. cornstarch
- 1 tsp. minced garlic
- 1 tsp. minced ginger
- 2 tbsp. avocado oil
- 1 ½ pound chicken breast
- Pinch of salt
- 1 tbsp. sesame seeds
- 2 tbsp. diced green onion
- 1 tbsp. sesame oil

In a bowl, start by whisking the ketchup, soy sauce, rice vinegar, cornstarch, garlic, and ginger. Set aside. Trim the fat from the chicken - cut into one-inch pieces. Heat avocado oil in a non-stick pan and add the chicken. Cook for 6-7 minutes, or until done. Next, add the sauce to the pan - cook for two additional minutes and transfer chicken to your plates, and top with sesame oil, sesame seeds, and green onion.

Creamy Keto Roasted Tomato Soup

Total Prep & Cook Time: 45 min.
Yields: 4 Servings

Ingredients:

- 10 Roma tomatoes, cut into cubes
- 4 garlic cloves
- 2 tbsp. olive oil
- 1 tbsp. Herbs of Provence
- ¼ c. heavy cream
- 2 c. chicken bone broth
- 2 tbsp. diced basil (fresh if possible)
- Pinch of salt

Preheat to reach 400 degrees Fahrenheit. Cover a baking tray using a layer of parchment baking paper. Toss the tomato pieces with olive oil and garlic and place them onto the baking sheet. Roast 25 minutes. (Alternatively, to save time, use one large can of roasted tomatoes.)

Transfer the tomato chunks into a blender or food processor, including the garlic and liquid, and blend until smooth. Return the mixture to the pot on the stove and add bone broth and herbs. Remove from heat and add heavy cream and diced basil. Serve.

Hearty Cheesy Mushroom Casserole

Total Prep & Cook Time: 45 min.
Yields: 4 Servings

Ingredients:

- 1 pound ground beef
- 1 pound mushrooms, sliced
- 5 cloves garlic, diced
- 8 slices Swiss cheese
- 1 c. crumbled goat cheese
- 1/3 c. scallions
- Pinch of salt
- Also Needed: 8x8 baking dish

Warm the oven to reach 375 degrees Fahrenheit. Next, prepare the baking dish by greasing it with olive oil or coconut oil. Add the beef and salt to a non-stick pan and heat on high until browned. Add mushrooms and garlic until liquid has evaporated (7-8 min.). Fold in goat cheese - plus half of the Swiss cheese until just melted. Transfer to a baking dish and top with scallions and remaining Swiss cheese. Bake uncovered for 10-15 minutes and you should serve it hot.

Tuna Zoodle Casserole

Total Prep & Cooking Time: 35 min.
Yields: 6 Servings

Ingredients:

- 3 zucchini, spiralized to become zoodles
- 1 tsp. diced garlic
- 1 tbsp. butter
- 1 c. unsweetened and unflavored almond milk
- ¼ c. heavy cream
- 1 c. shredded cheddar cheese
- 3 oz. cream cheese
- 1 can, 12-oz. tuna, drained
- Black pepper and salt (as desired)
- ½ c. additional cheddar cheese
- ½ c. mozzarella cheese

Set the oven temperature to reach 375 degrees Fahrenheit. Grease a big baking dish with olive oil or coconut oil. Place zoodles in the bottom of the dish. Bake zoodles at 10-minute intervals, stirring between intervals until done (approximately 20-30 minutes).

Melt butter in a medium non-stick skillet and add garlic, almond milk, heavy cream, and 1 cup of the cheddar cheese and the cream cheese. Whisk until smooth, then stir in the tuna. Pour this mixture into the baking dish on top of zoodles. Layer remaining cheese on top and bake for 20 minutes, or until bubbly. Serve hot.

Crispy Coconut Chicken Rolls

Total Prep & Cook Time: 25 min.
Yields: 4 Servings

Ingredients:

- 4 coconut wraps (found in natural grocery stores)

- 1 lb chicken thighs, boneless, cut into small cubes
- 3 tbsp. coconut oil
- 2 garlic cloves, diced
- 1/2 onion, diced
- 1 tbsp ginger
- 2 tsp. curry powder
- 2 tsp. smoked paprika
- 1/2 c. coconut milk
- ¼ c. chicken broth, unsweetened
- 2 tbsp. almond butter
- 2 tbsp. tomato paste
- 1 ½ c. cauliflower rice
- 1 c. baby spinach
- Pinch of salt

Warm the oil in a skillet. Cook the chicken, garlic, onion, ginger, salt, and pepper until the chicken is cooked through, or 5-8 minutes. Stir in the coconut milk, broth, almond butter, and tomato paste and simmer for 10 minutes.

In another skillet, cook the cauliflower rice with two tablespoons of water until done, approximately five minutes.

Spread out the coconut wraps and line with a layer of spinach. Distribute the chicken mixture and the cauliflower rice onto each wrap, then roll like a burrito. Serve warm or cold.

Keto Bacon Sushi Rolls

Total Prep & Cook Time: 25 min.
Yields: 4 Servings

Ingredients:

- 12 slices bacon
- ½ c. crab meat
- ½ c. avocado
- 2 tsp. sesame seeds

Preheat to 400 degrees. Lay the bacon strips on a piece of parchment paper on a baking tray - bake for 18 minutes, turning the bacon over once. Pat the cooked bacon dry of extra fat and roll the bacon into rolls (don't cook the bacon too crispy). Place the bacon rolls to the side to cool.

Unroll the cooked bacon once cool, and place a slice of avocado and 1-2 tsp. of crab meat onto one end. Re-roll the bacon, then sprinkle it with sesame seeds. You will be able to make 12 rolls of keto sushi.

Keto Charcuterie Board

Total Prep & Cook Time: 10 min.
Yields: 4 Servings

Ingredients:

- 2 triangles of brie
- 8 slices of cheddar or pepper jack cheese
- ½ c. goat or sheep cheese, spiced with Herbs of Provence
- ½ c. kalamata olives, warmed
- 8 slices of cured salami or pepperoni
- ½ c. sliced, roasted red bell pepper

Assemble the ingredients on a serving tray, serve as a side to any keto lunch for four people, or stand-alone lunch for two.

Steak Salad With Spicy Tarragon Dressing

Total Prep & Cooking Time: 20 min.
Yields: 4 Servings

Ingredients:

- 1/3 c. mayonnaise

- 2 tbsp. water
- ½ tbsp. dried tarragon
- ½ tbsp. Dijon mustard
- ½ tbsp. garlic powder
- 4 c. leafy greens
- 1 avocado, sliced
- 1 c. cherry tomatoes, halved
- 6 oz. cucumber
- 2 lbs. flank steak or rib-eye steak, cut into 1-inch pieces
- 2 tbsp. ghee or butter
- 2 garlic cloves

Whisk together the mayo, water, tarragon, mustard, and garlic powder, and refrigerate. Prep the greens and veggies and arrange in salad bowls. Warm the ghee or butter in a large non-stick skillet and cook the steak to your desired level of doneness. Season with salt and pepper.

Lay the steak cubes on top of your greens and veggies, and top with the refrigerated dressing.

Pulled Pork With Fire-Roasted Tomato Salad

Total Prep & Cook Time: 10 min.
Yields: 4 Servings

Ingredients:

- 2 lbs. pork shoulder
- 2 tbsp. olive oil
- 2 tbsp. cocoa nibs or cocoa powder
- ½ tsp. ginger
- ½ tbsp. paprika
- ½ tsp. cayenne pepper
- 4 c. leafy greens
- 2 c. cherry tomatoes, halved
- 3 tbsp. oil
- 1 tbsp. red wine vinegar
- 2 scallions
- 3 avocados
- ½ c. fresh cilantro
- ¼ c. lemon juice

Grind the spices and nibs and rub them on the pork shoulder. Slow cook the pork shoulder for six hours or until the meat can easily be shredded with a fork.

Alternatively, follow instructions for pressure cooking your pork roast.

To prepare the roasted tomato salad, roast tomatoes in the oven at 400 degrees after brushing with oil and lightly salting and peppering. Remove from your oven and place in a bowl with vinegar, oil, and scallions.

Make guacamole using avocados, lemon juice, and cilantro. Make a base with your pulled pork, and layer the tomato salad and guacamole on top. Serve with the pork warm or chilled.

Keto Dinner Recipes

Zucchini Keto Lasagna

Total Prep & Cooking Time: 45 min.
Yields: 6 Servings

Ingredients:

- 14 oz. zucchini, thinly sliced (use a slicer)
- 2 tbsp. olive oil
- 1 onion
- 2 garlic cloves/as desired
- 1 ½ pounds ground beef or ground turkey
- 1 tbsp. dried basil
- 1 tbsp. dried oregano
- 4 tbsp. tomato paste
- Salt and pepper to taste
- 1½ c. heavy whipping cream
- 3 tbsp. water
- 2 c. shredded cheese (mozzarella works best)

Set the oven temperature to reach 400 degrees. Slice the zucchini lengthwise with a vegetable slicer or peeler. Lay the zucchini slices on a paper towel to eliminate extra moisture, and then sprinkle with pepper and salt as desired.

Prepare the meat sauce by heating olive oil in a skillet using a medium-temperature setting. Dice and add the onion and garlic and cook until softened. Add the ground meat, basil, oregano, and more salt and pepper. Cook this mixture until it has browned, then stir in the tomato paste and the water - cook for five additional minutes.

Add the cream, half of the cheese, and the garlic to a different saucepan. Bring to a simmer until bubbling. Then reduce the temperature to medium-low. Simmer for five minutes.

Assemble the lasagna by layering the zucchini, the meat sauce, and the cheese sauce. Repeat layers until you've used all the ingredients. Top with remaining cheese and bake for 18-20 minutes.

Keto-Friendly Chicken Fajitas

Total Prep & Cook Time: 45 min.
Yields: 4 Servings

Ingredients:

- 1 ½ lbs. chicken breast, sliced into strips
- 2 cloves of garlic, diced
- 1 bell pepper, sliced
- 1 onion, sliced
- 1 tbsp. dried basil
- 1 tbsp. dried oregano
- 2 tsp. cumin
- 1 tbsp. chili powder
- 1 tbsp. paprika
- 1 tsp. salt
- ¼ c. olive oil or avocado oil
- Cilantro to garnish
- 2 avocados (for guacamole on the side)

Set the oven temperature to reach 400 degrees. Mix all the spices in a bowl. In a separate mixing container, toss the chicken and veggies with a drizzle of olive oil. Mix in the spice mix and stir to coat.

Pour the entire mixture onto a greased sheet pan and cook for 20 minutes, stirring a few times as necessary. Serve the fajita mix with guacamole, cilantro, and cheese, either on a bed of lettuce for a fajita salad or wrapped in an egg or coconut wrap for a fajita burrito.

Tex-Mex Beef Casserole

Total Prep & Cook Time: 35 min.
Yields: 4 Servings

Ingredients:

- 1 ½ lbs. ground beef or turkey
- 3 oz. butter or ghee
- 3 tbsp. Tex-Mex seasoning blend of your choice
- 1 c. crushed tomatoes
- 2 oz. pickled jalapenos
- 2 c. shredded cheddar cheese
- ¾ c. sour cream
- 6 oz. leafy greens
- 1 c. guacamole

Set the oven temperature to 400 degrees. You should fry the ground beef or ground turkey in butter using a medium-temperature setting in a non-stick pan until browned. Add the seasoning and tomatoes - simmer for five minutes.

Place the mixture in a greased baking dish and top with the jalapenos and cheese. Bake for 25 minutes and serve on a bed of leafy greens topped with sour cream and guacamole, as desired.

Baked Chicken With Cheesy Cauliflower Mash

Total Prep & Cook Time: 45 min.
Yields: 4 Servings

Ingredients:

- 2 lbs. chicken thighs, bone-in
- ¼ c. olive oil
- 3 tbsp. red wine vinegar
- ¼ c. lemon juice
- 2 tbsp. oregano
- 2 tbsp. thyme
- 2 garlic cloves, minced
- Black pepper and salt (as desired)
- 1 lb. cauliflower
- ¾ c. parmesan cheese
- 2 tbsp. olive oil
- 4 tbsp. butter or ghee

Whisk the olive oil with the lemon juice and spices in a ziplock bag. Add the chicken thighs to this marinade and toss to coat. Cover and seal and place in the refrigerator for three hours. Warm the oven to reach 400 degrees and cover a large baking tray with parchment paper. Bake the chicken for 35-40 minutes.

To make the cauliflower mash, slice the cauliflower into florets. Bring a pot of salted water to boil on the stove, and add in the cauliflower, boiling only until tender (just a few minutes). Drain your cauliflower and add to a food processor or blender, along with the butter and cheese. Blend until smooth (or desired consistency). Serve alongside the baked chicken.

Hearty Old-Fashioned Beef Stew

Total Prep & Cook Time: 60 minutes
Yields: 6 Servings

Ingredients:

- 2 lb. beef chuck roast or roast of choice, cut into cubes
- 2 tbsp. ghee
- 1 lb. radishes, trimmed and cut in half
- 6 ribs of celery, sliced
- 8 oz. mushrooms, sliced
- 6 c. beef bone broth
- 1 tbsp. cornstarch
- 1 tbsp. tomato paste
- 2 tbsp. oregano
- 2 tbsp. thyme
- 2 garlic minced cloves
- Black pepper and salt (to your liking)

Begin by seasoning the chuck roast with salt and pepper and set aside. Then, you should prep the radishes and celery. Mix the broth and the tomato paste in a small mixing container. Set this aside as well. In a large pot or Dutch oven, warm the ghee using a med-high temperature setting. Add the beef cubes to cover the pot (do not overlap beef). You should brown the beef for two minutes per side. Transfer it from the pot and place it on a layer of paper towels. Add another tablespoon of ghee to the pot and add the veggies and Italian seasonings and cook for three minutes or until softened. Pour the broth mixture into the pot or pan you have on hand

and add the meat. Bring to a simmer. Next, cook for 30 minutes.

Remove one cup of the broth and add the cornstarch. Redeposit this mixture back into the pot and cook for another 10 minutes.

Alternatively, follow your Instapot or other pressure cooker or slow cooker directions for preparing the stew.

Parmesan and Pecan-Encrusted Halibut

Total Prep & Cook Time: 45 min.
Yields: 2 Servings

Ingredients:

- 2 8-oz. halibut filets
- 2 tbsp. ghee or butter
- ¼ c. pecans
- ¼ c. parmesan cheese
- 2 tbsp. green onions, diced
- 1 tsp. minced garlic
- Juice from ½ lemon
- Black pepper and salt as desired

Combine the butter, pecans, parmesan, lemon juice, and garlic until blended.

Preheat the oven to 400 degrees. Dust the chicken using pepper and salt - bake for five minutes in a pan. Remove the pan from the oven and spread the topping over the fish. Bake until the fish is encrusted and the topping is crispy (10-12 min.).

Serve with zucchini zoodles or cauliflower rice on the side.

Keto Meatball and Mushroom Soup

Total Prep & Cooking Time: 45 min.
Yields: 4 Servings

Ingredients:

- 1 lb. ground Italian sausage
- 1 lb. ground pork
- ½ c. finely diced onion
- 1 stalk celery, diced
- 1 egg
- 1 additional onion, diced

- 2 tbsp. minced garlic
- 8 oz. cremini mushrooms, sliced
- 12 oz. beef stock or bone broth
- 2 large zucchini or yellow squash
- 2 additional stalks celery, sliced
- 1 tbsp. Italian herb seasoning
- 2 c. heavy whipping cream
- 1 c. grated parmesan cheese
- Salt and pepper to taste

Make the meatballs by combining the two meats, ½ c. onion, diced celery, and egg, and forming the mixture into 2-inch balls. Let this mixture of meatballs chill in the fridge for up to one hour.

Add olive oil to a large pan and add the meatballs, browning on all sides. Remove meatballs from the pan and set them on a paper towel. Using the same pan, add the onions, garlic, mushrooms, zucchini, and celery and brown until softened. This step should take about eight minutes.

Add the stock and meatballs, plus the Italian herbs. Allow the soup to simmer while the stock reduces, and then add in the cream and parmesan, whisking until well-combined. Serve the soup warm.

Shrimp With Creamy Cauliflower Grits

Total Prep & Cook Time: 25 min.
Yields: 4 Servings

Ingredients:

- 1 head of cauliflower
- 2 c. chicken broth or veggie broth
- 2 oz. cream cheese
- 1 c. shredded cheese of your choice
- 1 tbsp. butter or ghee
- 1 tbsp. minced garlic
- 3-4 tbsp. green onion
- 1 lb. deveined, peeled shrimp
- ½ tsp. paprika
- 1/8 tsp. red pepper flakes
- ¼ tsp. garlic powder
- 1 tbsp. Italian seasoning
- ¼ tsp. onion powder
- ¼ c. heavy cream
- Salt and pepper to taste

Make the grits using a medium-sized skillet or stock pan. Cut the cauliflower into florets, and bring the chicken stock to a boil. Add the florets and cook until tender.

Drain the broth and add the cream cheese, cheddar cheese, butter, salt, and pepper to the cauliflower. Mash until smooth (or until your desired consistency).

Make the shrimp by melting butter in a large skillet. Add the garlic and the shrimp, sprinkling with the Cajun spices. Stir well, so the spices are coating the shrimp, then cook for 3-4 minutes. Add the butter and also the heavy cream once the shrimp is pink and tender.

Divide the cauliflower grits between four bowls and top with the shrimp mixture. Garnish with green onion if desired.

Conclusion

Now that you're aware of the many benefits of a keto diet for women over 50 and realize that a keto diet doesn't have to be intimidating, it's time to get started on your own goals. You can use the previous chapters as a reference when you need reminders which foods are keto-friendly and on the no-go list and for inspiration for your keto shopping and cooking. You also now have health information and exercise plans at your fingertips.

As I said at the beginning of the book, as you begin to plan your keto diet, you will need a way to keep track of your macros, carbs, and calories and a place to organize your keto meal plan and weekly recipes.

Download the bundle and receive these completely free tools:

• A Daily Diet Tracker to keep track of the food you eat.

• A Daily Low Carb Tracker to keep track of the carbs you eat and you Carb Target.

- A Weekly Keto Meal Planner: We discussed the benefits of being prepared and having your keto menu planned out ahead of time. You will cheat fewer times and feel tempted less often! Our weekly planner has space for you to write down your keto meals for breakfast, lunch, and dinner every day for each week. Laminate this one-sheet planner and use a dry-erase marker to reuse it week by week, or simply print a new sheet every Sunday!

Here's the link to download them, copy it on your favorite device and enjoy!

https://www.subscribepage.com/ketodiettools

Thank you for making it through to the end of *Keto Diet for Women Over 50*. My goal for this guide was to provide a road map for other women over age 50 who wanted to make healthy changes and feel better every day. I hope this book has proven to be such a guide to you and that you now feel empowered to tackle your keto diet with confidence. I know you can find success!

If you found this a valuable book, a review on Amazon is always appreciated! I hope you will continue to leave new reviews as you continue on your keto journey, reach new goals, and gain new rewards.

Good luck, and remember that the resources you need are all at your fingertips.

Printed in Great Britain
by Amazon

75573558R00092